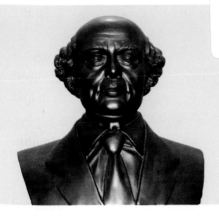

Dr. Samuel Hahnemann
The founder of Homoeopathy

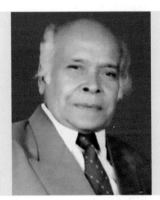

My Father philosopher guide
Late Dr. Dattatraya V. Nikam

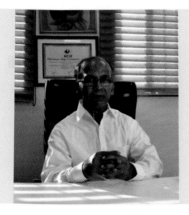

Dr.Amarsinha Nikam

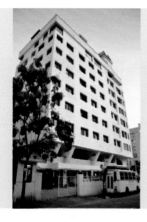

Hospital building with 100 bed facility

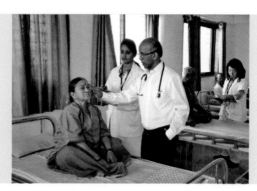

Hospital Round

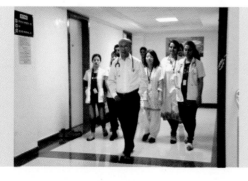

Doctors Team

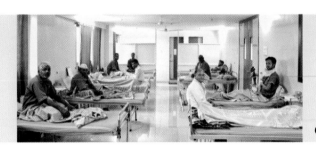

General ward

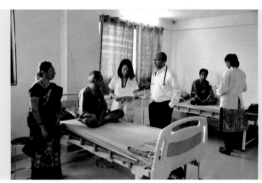

Semi Special ward

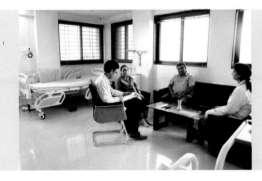

Delux Room

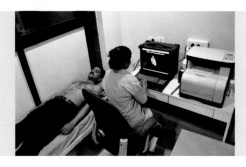

3 Dimensional
Cardiovascular
cartography machine

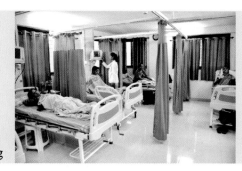

ICU Monitoring

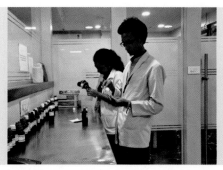

Aditya Homoeopathic
Hospital Pharmacy

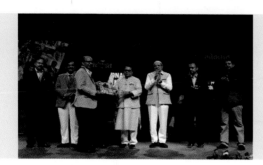

Dr. Nikam felicitated
with Lokmat Pune Icon
of the year

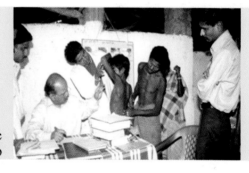

Free Homoeopathic
Medical camp

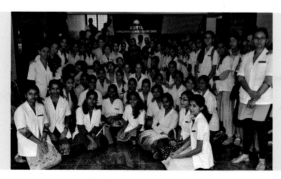

Frequent visits of
students to Aditya
Hospital

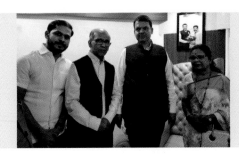

Dr. Nikam with The Honourable Devendra Fadnavis - Chief Minister of Maharashtra

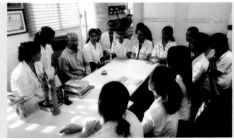

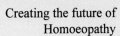

Creating the future of Homoeopathy

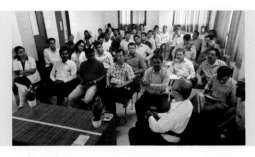

Classical Homeopathy Workshop

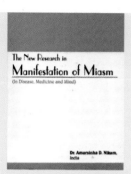

The New Research in
Manifestation of Miasm

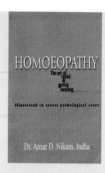

Homoeopathy The art of
rapid & gentle healing

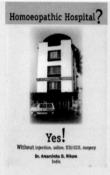

Homoeopathic Hospital

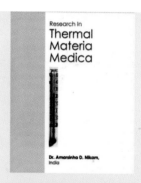

Thermal Materia Medica

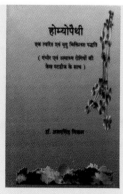

Homoeopathy in Hindi

Android Apps

Homoeo App
for every
Hompath
(Free)

Thermal Materia
Medica App ₹120/-

MISSION HOMOEOPATHY

Campaign to Save Classical Homoeopathy

Association for the Nurturing & Caring Classical Homoeopath

Founder chairman: Dr. Amarsinha D. Nikam.

About us

The association is the brain - child of Dr. Amarsinha D. Nikam. He is the shining example of the power and might of classical homoeopathy in the world.

Our Vision

- To create awareness about classical homoeopathy as a first choice of medical treatment in emergency, acute, sub-acute, chronic and curable life - threatening diseases.
- To help the oppressed and the downtrodden strata of society who absolutely cannot afford the traditional medical treatment.
- To save valuable natural resources and reduce the pollution.

Ongoing courses of the Association

- **For fresh graduates:** 6 months Residential training course at Aditya Homoeopathic Hospital.
- **For practitioners:** Classical Homoeopathy Workshop [6 sessions of 2 days in 1 year] A comprehensive training course which teach safe & successful way of treatment by adhering to classical methods.
- Seminar for spreading classical homoeopathy, Dr. Nikam continuously addresses the medical community to go for scientific & practical approach towards Homoeopathy at various places.
- Lectures and Social camp.

Vital Force
is
Oxygen

An Enlightening Research in Vital Force

Dr Amarsinha D. Nikam

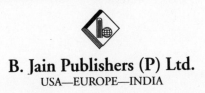

B. Jain Publishers (P) Ltd.
USA—EUROPE—INDIA

VITAL FORCE IS OXYGEN

First Edition: 2009
3rd Impression: 2018

Published by Kuldeep Jain for
B. JAIN PUBLISHERS (P) LTD.
D-157, Sector-63, NOIDA-201307, U.P. (INDIA)
Tel.: +91-120-4933333 • *Email:* info@bjain.com
Website: **www.bjain.com**
Registered office: 1921/10, Chuna Mandi, Paharganj,
New Delhi-110 055 (India)

Printed in India by
J.J. Offset Printers

ISBN: 978-81-319-0824-2

Dedicated to My Guru

−Dr Samuel Hahnemann

Preface

The vital force is an interesting concept of utmost importance in Homeopathic science. But, the theoretical rather an unscientific explanation of vital force was very confusing for homeopathic students and doctors.

The subject of vital force (vital energy) is a scientific and an important document of Homeopathy which was put forth by Master Hahnemann. But, it has been transformed into an unperceivable, an unexplainable, and an unscientific philosophy which has made homeopathic science a target for criticism in the medical world by other pathies.

Since, I was enrolled in first year in homeopathic college, I was eager to understand this interesting subject of vital force. But I was not being guided enthusiastically on this subject.

My father was a homeopathic consultant. I had seen the tremendous recovery and results. Since my childhood I had developed full faith on this science as I had been born and brought up with homeopathy. It compelled me to become a follower of this wonderful science. The keen interest for understanding the science kept me enthusiastic and my efforts helped me to perceive the concepts without any guidance.

After completing my college curriculum I continued with my study and practice. A continuous reading of Dr Hahnemann's philosophy and following his methods and principles of prescription gave me good results. This enhanced my knowledge and confidence in our pathy.

As I started practising, I came up with good results and witnessed amazing recoveries of patients. This success was giving me happiness. But, I wasn't satisfied with it, for me these results were of no use until they had a scientific explanation. This allowed other people to criticize me, call me a fluke and even a non-homeopathic method prescriber. This criticism made me aware of the truth and with acceptance I continued my journey.

I had done enormous readings of the books of Philosophies of our pioneers Dr Hahnemann, Dr Kent's, Dr H.A. Roberts and Dr Stuart Close and many more.

This brought me to a conclusion that 'Yes, our homeopathic philosophy has a solid scientific foundation!

Today, nearly after three decades of my practice, I have established an 80 beded homeopathic hospital which only works on a standard homeopathic prescription of 30 potency. Also, I have delivered many seminars through which I have put forth my classical and scientific way of homeopathic practice and understanding of homeopathic philosophy by different angles.

For the first time, I introduced this concept of vital force in 2005 at Singapore. The concept was greatly appreciated and the crowd was eager to know the subject in deep. This also inspired me to write a book on this concept.

To write a book was a very difficult task, I required a proper data to put forth my thoughts. This took me four years of hard & heart work to complete each matter in a scientific manner.

My only aim is to establish Homeopathy as a firm science; so that no one can ever criticize or underestimate it. To fulfill this purpose erasing the wrong concepts and inculcate the basic scientific concepts on the mind of newly emerging generation of Homeopaths is a necessity. It will strengthen their faith and dedication to the pathy.

This will result in wide spread of the pathy from richest to the commonest and to all corners of this world.

This book is a humble attempt made by me for better understanding and development of our pathy.

This is my request to the readers, take help of this book to make their concepts clearer regarding vital force and erase all the doubts in their mind; as in my previous books - 'The manifestation of Miasm' and 'Thermal Materia Medica'.

Dr Amarsinha D. Nikam

Acknowledgements

For the first time, I explored my deeper understanding of 'Vital Force' and shared my thoughts in the year 2005, at Singapore Seminar.

Dr Rangachari, the Principal of Singapore Homeopathic Faculty, and graduate and Post-Graduate students were astonished with my lecture on the Vital Force. Everybody appreciated and requested me to write a book on this scientific subject. That's why firstly I am expressing my sense of gratitude to all the students and especially Dr Rangachari.

Special thanks to Dr Rakhi Subhash Munot and Dr Neeta Kiran Jain who wrote down my delivered speech and helped me in writing this book. They have given me their precious time for writing this book. And my heartiest thanks to my daughter, Dr Suchitra and Dr Pallavi Bub for giving me full time support in completing this book.

I convey my heartiest thanks to my loving nephew Dr Rohit Deshmukh for helping and supporting me in every book.

It would not have been possible for me to complete the book within time, without the help of my students' (mentioned above) prompt and perfect work following action, under my guidance.

My special thanks to Dr Bharat B. Kale, who is Ph.D. (Scientist-E) who helped me with the scientific references. Also his student, Mr Yogesh Sonawane, who provided me the required and needed information.

My special thanks to Dr Vijay Satav, (M.D. Pathology), Chinchwad, Pune, who gave me valuable information about Pathology for this book.

All my thanks to my budding students Dr Sneha, Dr Sona and all my students and many budding students from B. V. P. Medical College, and other colleges whose great efforts made this task easy.

Difficult task of computerized formatting and composing of this book was done by Ms Vandana Kale by giving her valuable efforts to fulfill this task within time.

Special thanks to my close friend and colleague Dr Arun Jadhav, Principal, Bharati Vidyapeeth Homeo-pathic Medical College, Pune.

Mr Mahendra Konde, P.R.O. in my hospital who is always busy with Hospital activities and has always treasured the moments of special events by his excellent photography.

My mother who not only loves me but gives me encouragement, affection and blessings in every moment of my life.

Thanks to my wife, Sudha who is sacrificing her life for me and always encourages me in every moment of my life. She also gives attention towards Hospital Management and makes my task easy. My son Dr Vijaysinha and Dr Manish who helped me a lot for this book.

My brother, Mr Mahesh and his wife Mrs Rajashree look after my patients and are doing excellent service in Aditya Cafe.

My sisters and their family members always supported me in my mission.

My staff members who are tirelessly working day-night for my hospital in maintaining the rigors and serving my patients promptly to make this organization a unique picture of human service.

I want to thank lots of people who have always influenced and inspired me in my progressive work and whenever I remember them, I thank them in my heart.

Special Thanks and Gratitude

My special thanks to Hon.Cabinet Minister Mr Prithviraj Chauhan, Hon. Ex-Minister, Central Government, India, Mrs Suryakanta Patil, Mr Vilasrao Deshmukh (Heavy Industry, Cabinet Minister), Mr Govindrao Adik, Mr Vijaysinha Mohite-Patil, Mr Prataprao Bhosale and Mr Ulhasrao Pawar, Mr Sadakant (I.A.S. Joint Secretary, Home Ministry), Dr Patangrao Kadam (Hon. Minister, Maharashtra State), Mr Laxman Jagtap (M.L.A.), Mr Vilas Lande (M.L.A.), Mr Gajanan Babar (M.L.A.), Mr Prabhakar Deshmukh (Ex-Collector, Pune), Mr Gulabrao Pol (D.I.G. Police, Maharashtra State), Mr Dilip Band (Divisional Commissionar, Maharashtra State), Mr Anil Diggikar (Deputy-Comissionar, Mumbai) and Mr Pravinsinha Pardeshi (Ex-Commissionar, P.C.M.C. & Pune), Mr Shengaonkar, D.C.P., Pune (Commissioner Office)

My special thanks to Mr Shivajirao Kadam, Vice Chancellor of Bharati Vidyapeeth, Mr Uttamrao Bhoite (Executive Director) B. V. P, Pune, Mr S.F. Patil, Ex-Vice Chancellor, Principal Mr K. D. Jadhav, Director audit and Law, B. V.P. Pune.

My friend Mr Umeshchandra Upadhyay, Mr Umesh Chandgude (Social worker), Mr Hasan Tamboli (Industrialist, Satara), Mr Gaikwad Mama, Mr Amol Prabhu, Mr G. M. Mahale, Advocate Mr Mukundrao Awate.

My thanks to Principal and staff of Bharati Vidyapeeth Homeopathic Medical College, Pune, who honoured me with a post of Honorary Professor as well as Homeopathic Faculty member and encouraged me to share my work with budding Homeopaths.

Padmashree Dr D.Y. Patil and Mrs Patil (D.Y. Patil University), and Mr Arun Chopra, Ex-Comd. N.D.A., always inspire me.

Dr Mrs Dehalani Madam, Vice Principal, Foster Hom. Med. College, Aurangabad.

I.I.H.P. (Mumbai) the biggest group of classical Homeopathy taking tremendous efforts to spread Homeopathy in practitioners and students, always invited me every year to conduct a Seminar on Homeopathy.

'Study Circle Group' from Mumbai which is also popular among the practitioners and students, conducting lots of my Seminars at Mumbai to share my experiences in Homeopathy.

UHA, Classical Homeopathic Group from Nagpur – Dr Ashish, Dr Shilpa, Dr Yadnik and other students who are doing good work for spreading Classical Homeopathy.

To various Homeopathic colleges from all over India which have regularly invited me to deliver a speech on Classical Homeopathy and Homeopathic Hospital practice.

Editor of 'Homeopathic Community Journal' Dr Neelam Avtar Singh and Association for Scientific

Research in Homeopathy Group who arranged my seminar at Patiala – Dr Amar Singh Maan, Dr Avtar Singh and Dr H.S. Matharoo who comes all the way from Punjab to observe Classical Homeopathic work at my hospital.

Editor of 'Homeopathic Mind Journals' Dr Ashok Gupta, who always spends his valuable time for me, writing articles on my hospital cases. Now, he is enjoying Classical Homeopathy at Baithia, Bihar. He has also arranged video seminar of my cases at Bihar.

The Organizer of 'The Research Society of Homeopathy' – Dr C.P.Singh, Dr Anurudh Verma, Dr Jitendra Verma and other students from U.P. who invited me for - National Seminar on Applied Homeopathy at Lucknow.

I would also like to forward my gratitude to the editor of H-pathy Dr. Manish Bhatia.

I also thank my friends Mr Faizy Dalal and Mr Lalit Fulfagar for bringing critical cases to me.

I am also thankful to B. Jain Publishers, Dr. Geeta Rani Arora and all editorial staff of B. Jain Publishers.

Contents

Introduction

Introduction

'Homeopathy' is a science which is based on the philosophy of Dr Samuel Hahnemann the pioneer of homeopathy, who was not only a scientist but also a great philosopher. His concept about the foundation on which he put forth the homeopathic principles like 'Similia Similibus Curentur' is very crystal clear but very few classical homeopaths really understand them. The same thing happened with Hahnemann's book of Homeopathic philosophy i.e. 'The Book of Organon of Medicine'.

According to me, the law of 'Similia Similibus Curentur' means:

Similia: It means similar symptoms (with similar character with similar constitution and similar thermals).

Similibus: It means exact miasm which means exact degree of pathology that should be matched with medicinal manifestation of symptoms.

Curentur: If the patient's symptoms are exactly matching with the symptoms of medicine, then only cure will be possible.

There are ample misconceptions about Homeopathic philosophy & everyone tries to analyze and apply this philosophy according to their intelligence and understanding. It ends up in varied theories & concepts which create confusion amongst homeopaths. There are different ways of understanding homeopathic concepts, which is also seen, in terms of miasms.

Many homeopaths face a common difficulty of how to understand the concept of miasms (Psora, Sycosis, Tybercular and Syphilis). Once you are aware of manifestations of miasm, only then you will find out similar picture which exactly matches with the diseased picture, this will be possible only after following the basic laws & principles of the pathy. The miasm and the constitution that is physical and mental makeup of an individual, for example: his desires, adversions, modalities, thirst, body discharges & also the thermal sensitivity (that is sensitivity to heat & cold) along with patient's mental state should be taken into consideration while prescribing. Everyone should follow this simple principle at every step of case taking and prescribing.

But unfortunately some homeopaths prescribe according to pathology and diseased state without understanding the concept of miasm. Some are prescribing the medicine according to the particular organ or gland affection (organ/specific remedy). Also there is a trend in newly growing homeopaths that without understanding the constitution and manifestation of miasm, they treat only relying on mental state. The mental state does not depict the exact constitution of a sick person as it will not guide the exact physical sensations, symptoms, thermal state, clinical parameters of the patient and also the gravity of disease state. Hence the 'Law of Similar' is not going to be followed; definitely the result will not be satisfactory and the cure will be impossible. Thus, every homeopath should follow the basic principles & philosophy behind the prescription.

While explaining the homeopathic philosophy, Dr Hahnemann introduced the most important concept 'Vital Force' and its role in human body' in which he noted precisely that Vital Force is centrally and universally acting on each & every human being. The whole disease concept is dependent on the derangement of the Vital Force, as it is the central and dynamic force which governs all over the body from the most important organs up to the basic cellular level.

Dr Hahnemann mentioned about the concept of Vital Force in organon that – derangement of Vital Force is the root cause of all the diseases. So every physician should try restoring the health by removing the disturbance which occurred on the Vital Force and attain cure. But, the followers of this pathy do not know what exactly it is? Since last 200 long years we were in dark. Due to lack of knowledge and understanding no one tried to analyse Dr Hahnemann's concept of Vital Force or dynamic force. I think there is still a great confusion regarding this concept.

In this book, I would like to introduce a clear concept of Vital Force by **scientific way** which will be easily acceptable to the modern science and they will thus accept the Hahnemannian thoughts behind this philosophy. Obviously, it will be helpful for every homeopathic student and they will be proud about Hahnemannian philosophical thoughts which were truly based on nature's law and now are correlated scientifically.

This book is an attempt to convey the role of vital force in human life by proving it scientifically.

Before reading this book please be thorough with the basics of cell's, structure, function and metabolism of foodstuffs.

CHAPTER 2

Different Concepts of Vital Force

APHORISMS RELATED TO VITAL FORCE

CONCEPT BY DR KENT – SIMPLE SUBSTANCE

CONCEPT BY DR HERBERT ROBERTS

CONCEPT BY STUART CLOSE – VITAL PRINCIPLE

CONCEPT BY VITHOULKAS – CONCEPT OF RESONANCE, ELECTRO-DYNAMIC FIELD

Different Concepts of Vital Force

There are many mysterious thoughts in homeopathy regarding the concept of vital force. Even the homeopathic stalwart could not come to the clear conclusion of realistic and scientific definition of vital force. Due to this mysterious circle, vital force remained in dark and this being a query no one could prove it scientifically. As a result, the homeopathic students, practitioners, and consultants are highly puzzled regarding this concept. This is one of the reasons for other medical sciences to criticize homeopathy regarding this notion. There is a stigma on homeopathy that it is not a scientific, but an imaginary science.

When Dr Samuel Hahnemann discovered homeopathy, modern science was in dark. It was a great appreciable thing that with few limited resources he arrived at the concept of vital force. At his time, there was lack of equipments and technical help; but with the clinical knowledge and deep study about human health, life, and sickness this master minded man tried to prove Homeopathy as a perfect and fundamental science.

There were four epochal in the history of practice of medicine, the first one Hippocrates, the great observer who introduced the art of clinical observation for pathological diagnosis. Second, Galen, the disseminator, who spread the teachings of Hippocrates over the medical world. Third, is Paracelsus, who introduced physical as well as chemical analysis in Practice of Medicine. Fourth, Dr Hahnemann, whose experimental mind discovered the symptomatic source of both pathological and therapeutic diagnosis and thereby made practice of medicine scientific. At the same time he explained that vital force plays an important role for healthy and harmonious life.

APHORISMS RELATED TO VITAL FORCE

In aphorism 9 of 'Organon of Medicine', he mentioned that 'In the healthy condition of man, the spiritual vital force (autocracy), the dynamis that animates the material body (organism), rules with unbounded sway, and retains all the parts of the organism in admirable, harmonious, vital operation, as regards both sensations and functions, so that our indwelling, reason gifted mind can freely employ this living, healthy instrument for the higher purposes of our existence.'

In aphorism 10 'The material organism, without the vital force, is capable of no sensation, no function, no self preservation; it derives all sensation and performs all the functions of life solely by means of the immaterial being (the vital principle) which animates the material organism in health and in disease.'

In aphorism 11 of Organon, he mentioned that 'When a person falls ill, it is only this spiritual, self acting (automatic) vital force, everywhere present in his organism, that is primarily deranged by the dynamic influence upon it of a morbific agent inimical to life; it is only the vital principle, deranged to such an abnormal state, that can furnish the organism with its disagreeable sensations, and incline it to the irregular processes which we call disease; for, as a power invisible in itself, and only cognizable by its effects on the organism, its morbid derangement only makes itself known by the manifestation of disease in the sensations and functions of those parts of the organism exposed to the senses of the observer and physician, that is, by morbid symptoms, and in no other way can it make itself known.'

CONCEPT BY DR KENT – SIMPLE SUBSTANCE

In 'Kent's Lectures on Homeopathic Philosophy', a chapter on simple substance, Dr Kent had mentioned that if Dr Hahnemann might had used the word immaterial vital substance, it would have been even stronger, for you will see it to be true that it is a substance...

Dr Kent says further in this chapter that, at the present day advanced thinkers are speaking of the fourth state of matter which is immaterial substance. We now say the solids, liquids, and gases and the radiant form of matter. Substance in simple form is just as positively substance as matter in concrete form. The question then comes up for consideration and study: What is the vital force? What is its character, quality, or essence? For a number of years there has been a continuous discussion of force as force, or power to construct. If man can think of energy as something substantial he can better think of something substantial as having energy. He must think in a series whereby cause enters into effect and furthermore into a series of effects. If he does not do this he destroys the very nature and idea of influx and continuance. If man does not know what is continuous, if he does not realize that there are beginnings, intermediates and ends, he cannot think, for the very foundation of the thought is destroyed.

The materialist to be consistent with his principles is obliged to deny the soul, and to deny a substantial God, because the energy which he dwells upon so much is nothing, and he must assume that God is nothing, and therefore there is none. But the one who is rational will be led to see that there is a supreme God, that He is substantial, that he is a substance. Everything proceeds from him and the whole series from the supreme to the most ultimate matter in this way is connected.

There are many qualities predicated of simple substance.

1. One of the first propositions we have to consider is that - Simple substance is endowed with formative intelligence, i.e., it intelligently operates and forms the economy of the whole animal, vegetable, and mineral kingdoms. The simple substance gives to everything its own type of life, gives it distinction, and gives it identity whereby it differs from all other things. This is due to the formative intelligence of simple substances.

2. This substance is subject to changes, i.e. it may be in order or disordered. It may be normal or sick.

3. Any simple substance may pervade the entire material substance without disturbing or replacing it.

4. When the simple substance is an active substance it dominates and controls the body, it occupies. It is the cause of force. The body does not move, think, or act unless it has its interior degrees of immaterial substance, which acts upon the economy continuously in the most beautiful manner, but as soon as the body is separated from its characterizing simple substance there is a cessation of influx. The energy derived from the simple substance keeps all things in order. By it are kept in order all functions, and the perpetuation of the forms and proportions of every animal, plant, and mineral. All operation that is possible is due to the simple substance, and by it the very universe itself is kept in order.

5. Matter is subject to reduction, and it can be continuously reduced until it is in the form of simple substance, but it is not subject to restitution.

6. The simple substances may exist as simple, compound or complex, and as such never disturb harmony, but always continue from first to last, and in that way all purposes are conserved.

7. Dynamic simple substances often dominate each other in proportion to their purpose, one having a higher purpose than another. This vital force, which is a simple substance, is again dominated by another simple substance still higher, which is the soul.

8. Simple substances are not subject to physical law. In considering simple substance we can't think of time, place, space, weight, or gravity.

9. Quantity cannot be predicted of simple substance; only quality in degrees of fineness can be predicted.

10. The simple substance also has adaptation. The simple

substance when it exists in the living human body keeps that body animated, keeps it moving, perfects its uses, superintends all parts and at the same time keeps the operation of mind and will in order.

11. We see also that this vital substance when in a natural state, when in contact with the human body, is constructive; it keeps the body continuously constructed and reconstructed. When these forces are not dominated and controlled by the vital force the body tends to decay at once. So we see that the vital force is constructive or formative, and in its absence there is death and destruction.

CONCEPT BY DR HERBERT ROBERTS

Dr Herbert Roberts the stalwart of homeopathy writes in his book 'The Principles and Art of Cure by Homeopathy'; in 3rd chapter of vital force that

'When the two parent cells are united that vital principle, the vital energy, is already present; and the ego of the completed cell does not change one iota after once beginning its process; it has in itself and of itself the power to develop the cells, the physical, because of the continual flowing through them of the vital energy which dominates the whole. It has within itself the power to develop muscle, nerve, brain – cells individual in themselves, gifted with the powers for specialized uses in the future. Without this vital energy, the cell, or the whole body, becomes inanimate and is dead. It is only when the vital energy is present that there is a living organism, capable of physical action and of the exercise of mental powers and the ability to take hold on the spiritual forces.

The nature of energy is dynamic, and this dynamis penetrates every particle, every cell, and every atom of the human economy.

Any disturbance of this vital energy or force results in a disfigured or disturbed development of the whole human economy. Such a disturbance may come from pre-natal influences, such as the effects of sudden fright; it may be caused by indulgences on the part of either or both parents at the time of conception; the cause may lie in excessive worry during gestation; it may be due to hereditary stigma of either one or both of the parent cells, which may perhaps be due to hereditary diseases or miasms. On the other hand, after the separate individual life has been established, we know how terrific the consequences of fright are. It transmits the effects to the vital energy long after the incident is forgotten. These are but a few instances where there may be serious disturbances of the vital force.

The influence of this vital force on the whole organism is so delicately adjusted and so intimately connected with every part, that seemingly distant organs or unrelated symptoms show the effects of any disturbance of the vital force.

The appearance of these disturbances is a reflection of the inward turmoil and confusion of the harmonious action which the vital force has suffered.

CONCEPT BY STUART CLOSE – VITAL PRINCIPLE

Stuart Close in his book 'The Genius of Homeopathy' writes about vital force that:

Vital Principle governs the vital energy to liberate vital force within special type of atoms and then –

Atoms are combined in different ways to yield the monomers (amino acids, nucleotides, and sugar) which are the building blocks of biological macromolecules (proteins, nucleic acids, polysaccharides). Macromolecules are combined with smaller molecule to form cell organelles (the cell membrane, mitochondria, lysosomes, and endoplasmic reticulum). The organelles are combined to form cells, the cells to form tissue, the tissue to form organs and the organs to form organism.

In this way modified universal energy (vital force) works in the living body for the higher purpose of our existence.

From the language of Stuart Close we can quote again:

'Everything living comes from preceding life in an unbroken chain, the last conceivable link of which is in the one infinite and eternal source of life, the Supreme Being. Metaphysical science recognizes this conception under the term of 'The Cosmic Life'.

Motion is the result of the application of force. Force is the product of power or energy.

All reactions to stimuli by which the functions and activities of the living body are carried on, originate in the primitive life substance at the point where it becomes materialized as cells and protoplasmic substance.

The phenomena of life, as manifested in growth, nutrition, repair, secretion, excretion, self-recognition, self-preservation, and reproduction, all take their direction from an originating center. From the lowest cell to the highest and most complex organism, this principle holds true. Cell wall and protoplasmic contents develop from the central nucleus and that from the centrosome, which is regarded as the 'center of force' in the cell. All fluids, tissues, and organs develop from the cell from within outwards, from center to circumference.

Organic control is from the center. In the completely developed human organism vital action is controlled from the central nervous system. The activities of the cell are controlled from the centrosome, which may be called the brain of the cell.

How or by what else could the vital force necessary to carry on vital processes be generated? How else could there be in the cell a 'dynamic center'? Dynamic center means 'center of power'. Statically, power means capacity of a person or thing for work, for producing the force by which work is done. There must be a source from which force is produced or drawn, and that source must be substantial. Kinetically, power is the cause, force the medium, and work the effect.

It is an axiom of biological science that life comes only from preceding life.

The central nervous system, made up of innumerable cells, with their nuclei and centrosomes, has already been compared to a dynamo. So each individual cell with its nucleus and centrosome may be called a dynamo in miniature. A dynamo is essentially a converter of one form of energy into another. Standing at the center of the field of attraction and acting in all directions under the law of attraction, the centrosome, through the agency of induction from the surrounding vital field, converts the chemical energy derived from nutrient matter into vital energy.....

CONCEPT BY VITHOULKAS – CONCEPT OF RESONANCE, ELECTRO-DYNAMIC FIELD

George Vithoulkas in his book 'The Science of Homeopathy' mentioned that everything in the universe, life itself is dependent on energy and on action and reaction. With decreasing life-energy, life itself dies. We therefore can hypothesize that the vital force is synonymous with the electro-dynamic field of the body and therefore confirms to known principles of physics.

Matter and energy interchange in the electro-dynamic field. This field is measurable in terms of waveforms, composed of frequency, wavelength, and amplitude. This is a given fact by laws of physics.

Now if everything in the universe vibrates at its own frequency, this also means the vital force, the electro-dynamic field of a living body, has to vibrate at its own frequency too. Important to know is, that though every substance vibrates at its own frequency, the vibration will increase when stimulated by a similar frequency. This shows that vibration even from a distance has an effect but the similar vibration is the more harmonious and stronger.

But what does that mean for homeopathy and for the vital force? The vital force is electro-dynamic energy, as we know. Therefore, it has its own frequency of vibration, though much more complex as the vibration of a non-homogenous substance. Because it affects all levels of the being at once and it has to respond on all influences of the environment and surroundings, it has to be able to change from moment to moment in frequency, regularity, and amplitude as well. That's what we call the 'Concept of Resonance'.

The vital force has to respond and adjust on every stimulus it is exposed to. The vital force can respond and adjust easily and unnoticeably to most minor stimuli we are exposed to in daily life. If however, the strength of stimulus is stronger than the vital force itself, it is forced to adjust in such a way, that the consequences are now perceivable by the trinity of body, mind, and spirit, depending on the adaptation of the vital force, more noticeable in body, mind, or spirit. This phenomenon Vithoulkas calls the 'Defense Mechanism', because if the vital force wouldn't adjust to these stimuli (these foreign vibration frequencies), the order in the body would soon get out of balance and inevitably, the body would die.

The concept of resonance clearly shows that every stimulus has an affect on the vital force and it either can adjust or respond to it without remarkable symptoms or with remarkable symptoms – depending on whether the stimulus is stronger or weaker than the vital force itself. Thus, the electro-magnetic field, the vital force, can be brought back into balance.

Oxygen

Oxygen

Oxygen is derived from the Greek word, where *oxys* means acid, literally sharp from the taste of acids and *genes* means producer, literally begetter. It is the element with atomic number 8 and represented by the symbol 'O'. It is a highly reactive non-metallic period 2 element that readily forms compounds (notably oxides) with almost all other elements. Oxygen is the third most abundant element in the universe by mass after hydrogen and helium. Diatomic oxygen gas constitutes 21% of the volume of air. Water is the most familiar oxygen compound.

OXYGEN HISTORY

Oxygen makes up 21% of the atmosphere we breathe, but it was not discovered as a separate gas until the late 18th century. Oxygen was independently discovered by Carl Wilhelm Scheele, in Uppsala in 1773 or earlier and by Joseph Priestley in Wiltshire, in 1774. The name oxygen was coined in 1777 by Antoine Lavoisier.

Although oxygen plays a life-supporting role, it took

about 150 years for the gas to be used in a proper manner for patients. After this discovery, therapeutic use of oxygen was only occasional or rare. The oxygen therapy was placed on a rational, scientific basis and was being used in the 20th century.

18ᵗʰ Century

- 1783 – Caillens: First case in which oxygen actually employed as a remedy (as quoted by Smith).

19ᵗʰ Century

- 1820 – Hill: Practical observations on the use of oxygen, or vital air in the cure of diseases.
- 1857 – Birch: On the therapeutic use of oxygen.
- 1869 – Mackey: On the therapeutical value of the inhalation of oxygen gas.
- 1870 – Barth: Oxygen: A remedy in disease.
- 1870 – Smith: Oxygen gas as a remedy in disease.
- 1872 – Davenport: Oxygen as a remedial agent.
- 1886 – Wallian: A further word on oxygen treatment and oxygen charlatans.
- 1886 – Smith: Clinical notes: Oxygen in therapeutics.
- 1887 – Osler: The treatment of pneumonia.
- 1888 – Kellogg: Oxygen enemata as a remedy in certain diseases.

20ᵗʰ Century

- 1908 – Bainbridge: Oxygen in medicine and surgery.
- 1912 – Hill: The administration of oxygen.

- 1914 – Howitt: The subcutaneous injection of oxygen gas.
- 1916 – Tunnicliff & Stebbing: The intravenous injection of oxygen gas.
- 1917 – Haldane: The therapeutic administration of oxygen.
- 1917 – Meltzer: The therapeutic value of oral rhythmic insufflation of oxygen.
- 1920 – Haldane & Barcroft: Oxygen' therapy.
- 1922 – Haldane: Respiration.
- 1928 – Cunningham: 'Monster Steel Ball' hyperbaric chamber.

STRUCTURE

At standard temperature and pressure, oxygen is a colourless, odorless gas with the molecular formula O_2 in which the two oxygen atoms are chemically bonded to each other with a spin triplet electron configuration.

PHYSICAL PROPERTIES

Oxygen is soluble in water. Oxygen condenses at 90.20 K (-182.95°C, - 297.31°F) and freezes at 54.36 K (-218.79°C, -361.82 °F)

It is a highly reactive substance.

Oxygen is artificially produced by fractional distillation of liquefied air, use of zeolites to remove carbon dioxide and nitrogen from air, electrolysis of water and other means. Oxygen exists in three forms solid, liquid, and gaseous form. Liquid oxygen is pale blue in colour.

OCCURRENCE

Oxygen is the most abundant chemical element by mass, in our biosphere, air, sea, and land. Earth is unusual among the planets of the solar system in having such a high concentration of oxygen gas in its atmosphere.

The unusually high concentration of oxygen gas on earth is the result of the oxygen cycle. This biogeochemical cycle describes the movement of oxygen within and between its three main reservoirs on earth that is the atmosphere, the biosphere and the lithosphere. The main driving factor of the oxygen cycle is photosynthesis, which is responsible for modern earth's atmosphere. Photosynthesis releases oxygen into the atmosphere, while respiration and decay remove it from the atmosphere.

BIOLOGICAL ROLE

The molecular dioxygen (O_2) is essential for cellular respiration in all aerobic organisms. Oxygen is used in mitochondria to generate adenosine triphosphate (ATP) during oxidative phosphorylation. The oxygen remaining after oxidation of the water molecule is released into the atmosphere.

ALLOTROPES OF OXYGEN

There are several known allotropes of oxygen.

1. Dioxygen, O_2 - Colourless

2. Ozone, O_3 - Blue

3. Tetraoxygen, O_4 - Metastable

4. Solid oxygen exists in six variously coloured phases - of which one is O_8 and another one metallic.

Dioxygen

The common allotrope of elemental oxygen on earth, O2, is known as dioxygen. Elemental oxygen is most commonly encountered in this form, as about 21% (by volume) of Earth's atmosphere.

Singlet oxygen

Singlet oxygen is the common name used for the two metastable states of molecular oxygen (O2) with higher energy than the ground state triplet oxygen.

Ozone

Triatomic oxygen (Ozone, O3), is a very reactive allotrope of oxygen that is destructive to materials like rubber and fabrics and is also damaging to lung tissue. Traces of it can be detected as a sharp, chlorine-like smell coming from electric motors, laser printers, and photocopiers.

Ozone is thermodynamically unstable towards the more common dioxygen form, and is formed by reaction of O2 with atomic oxygen produced by splitting of O2 by UV radiation in the upper atmosphere. Ozone absorbs strongly the ultraviolet rays and functions as a shield for the biosphere against the mutagenic and other damaging effects of solar UV radiation. Ozone is formed near the earth's surface by the photochemical disintegration of nitrogen dioxide from the exhaust of automobiles. Ground-level ozone is an air pollutant that is especially harmful for senior citizens, children, and people with heart and lung conditions such as

Emphysema, Bronchitis, and Asthma. The immune system produces ozone as an antimicrobial. Liquid and solid O_3 have a deeper-blue colour than ordinary oxygen and they are unstable and explosive.

Electrical discharges cause dioxygen to split into oxygen radicals. Most of these recombine to form dioxygen, but a few react with dioxygen to give ozone:

$$O_2 + O \rightarrow O_3$$

The ozone molecules themselves can also react with oxygen free radicals, to reform dioxygen, and so the actual concentration of atmospheric ozone is quite small. It is believed that ozone is formed in the upper atmosphere by the photo dissociation of dioxygen by the intense ultraviolet radiation from the sun. This light energy is thus absorbed; otherwise it would reach the Earth and destroy all life quite rapidly. Ozone is a greenhouse gas and, as such, would contribute to global warming if present in the lower atmosphere.

Tetraoxygen

Tetraoxygen had been suspected to exist since the early 1900, when it was known as oxozone, and was identified in 2001. The molecule O_4 was thought to be in one of the phases of solid oxygen later identified as O_8.

ISOTOPES

Planetary geologists have measured different abundances of oxygen isotopes in samples from the earth, the moon, mars, and meteorites. Analysis of a silicon wafer exposed to solar wind in space has shown that the sun has a higher proportion of oxygen-16 than does the earth. Also oxygen-16 is synthesized at the end of the helium fusion process in stars.

OXIDES AND OTHER INORGANIC COMPOUNDS

Many minerals for example, Calcium Carbonate ($CaCO_3$) require oxygen for formation of compounds (oxidation) and also for completion of their atomic structure by ion binding (oxidation).

Oxygen as a compound is present in the atmosphere in trace quantities in the form of carbon dioxide.

The earth's crustal rock is composed in large part of oxides of silicon, aluminium and other metals. The rest of the earth's crust is also made of oxygen compounds, in particular calcium carbonate and silicates.

Oxygen Energy is Nothing but the Vital Energy

Oxygen Energy is Nothing but the Vital Energy

Presence of oxygen marks existence of life in the whole universe. There will be no living organisms who can survive without this vital energy. Even the sun and the stars will not shine without this vital fuel. Along with oxygen, helium and hydrogen are also responsible for the sun's brightness. Even moon and few planets are said to contain solid form of oxygen. Whenever the presence of oxygen is less or zero it will lead to destruction. Earth became alive due to this vital energy (that is oxygen). Three fourth part of earth contains sea water (H_2O). Evaporation of water converts into clouds which contain hydrogen & oxygen. These clouds carry million litres of water to shower rain on the earth and thus recycling the vital energy which is useful for living organisms, on earth (including plants and animals) and in sea (marine plants and animals). Sea plants and animals utilize oxygen in liquid form.

Atmospheric fresh oxygen is absorbed by respiration. If there is any hindrance in the oxygen supply even for few minutes, the organism would be unable to sustain life. Thus, in every moment it plays a vital role in living organism as in functions and sensations which cannot be carried without oxygen. Even for the anaerobic organisms the combination of oxygen with carbon that is carbon dioxide is essential, for example, marine plant like green algae and cyanobacterium utilize carbon dioxide for their survival.

All major classes of structural molecules in living organisms, such as proteins, carbohydrates and fats, contain oxygen, as do the major inorganic compounds that comprise animal shells, teeth, and bone.

As everybody knows that plants are one of the source of oxygen; they use carbon dioxide for their food and release oxygen energy, which is utilized by human beings and animals. Presence of oxygen marks the survival of human being on the earth.

Its other application includes its utility for combustion (e.g. burning of a candle, etc.) and in solid form for combustion as in the rocket fuel (hydrogen, oxygen, and nitrogen) as well as in industries. Thus, Oxygen proves to be an oxidant and a vital fuel.

Above description proves universal requirement of oxygen.

CHAPTER 5

How the Vital Force (Oxygen) enters the Human Body?

RESPIRATORY SYSTEM

EXCHANGE OF RESPIRATORY GASES BETWEEN BLOOD AND ALVEOLI

DIFFUSION OF OXYGEN

- From atmophere to the alveoli
- From alveoli into the blood
- Diffusion of oxygen from blood into the tissues

TRANSPORT OF OXYGEN IN BLOOD

- As simple physical solution
- In combination with haemoglobin

ROLE OF OXYGEN IN RESPIRATORY CONTROL

How the Vital Force (Oxygen) enters the Human Body?

The founder of Homeopathy Samuel Hahnemann had given explanation of vital force in his book of Organon. Till date the stalwarts of homeopathy also couldn't come to the ultimate scientific conclusion as what vital force really is? How vital force enters in our body? Which activities take place in our body during the metabolism and to how this vital force is essential for every fraction of second for cellular metabolism and activities?

When the fresh air is taken through the nostrils it enters the lung and fills it with air which is rich in oxygen. The molecules of oxygen then pass through the airway into the thin wall of alveoli to the lungs and enter into the blood (i.e. diffusion). Here, it attaches itself to the haemoglobin in the blood and heart pumps the oxygenated blood to all the parts of our body. Haemoglobin then releases the oxygen so that it can reach to each and every cell of the body and this is how the vital energy, the vital force or the oxygen energy works. It gives energy and life itself.

Let us see how oxygen works in our body.

The **respiratory system** of every organism is responsible for oxygen exchange in it.

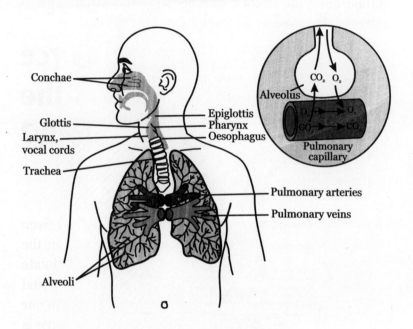

Fig.: 5.1 – Respiratory Passages

Respiration occurs in two stages, inspiration, and expiration. Exchange of respiratory gases i.e. oxygen and carbon dioxide between alveoli of the lungs and blood is called external respiration and, the exchange of gases between blood and the tissues is called internal respiration.

Exchange of respiratory gases between blood and alveoli

Respiratory unit is the terminal portion of respiratory tract and the exchange of gases between blood and atmospheric air occurs only in this part of the respiratory tract. The respiratory unit includes respiratory bronchioles, alveolar ducts, atria, alveolar sacs, and alveoli.

During inspiration when air enters the lungs, oxygen is diffused into the alveolar air constantly and carbon dioxide diffuses into alveolar air from pulmonary blood.

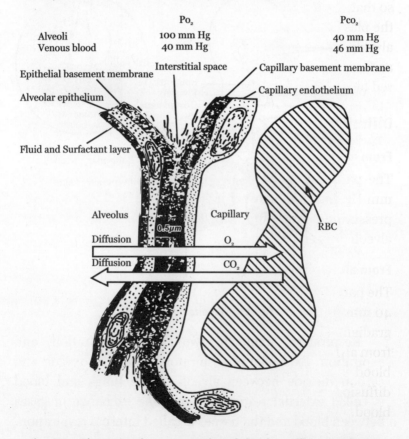

Fig.: 5.2 – **Diagrammatic representation of alveolo-capillary membrane showing the O_2 diffusion from the surfactant layer ⟶ alveolar epithelial cell cytoplasm ⟶ capillary basement membrane ⟶ endothelial cell cytoplasm ⟶ plasma. The CO_2 diffuses reversely.**

Respiratory membrane which is formed by the epithelium of the respiratory unit and endothelium of pulmonary capillaries plays a prime role in exchange of respiratory gases. The average diameter of pulmonary capillary is of eight microns which means that red blood cells squeeze through the capillaries. Therefore, the membrane of red blood cells is actually having contact with capillary wall so that, the oxygen or carbon dioxide need not pass through the plasma, while diffusing between the red blood cells and alveoli. Thus oxygen can easily enter into the red blood cells and, carbon dioxide can easily enter into the alveoli from the red blood cells.

Diffusion of oxygen

From atmosphere to the alveoli

The partial pressure of oxygen in the atmosphere is 159 mm Hg and in the alveoli it is 104 mm Hg. Because of the pressure gradient of 55 mm Hg, oxygen easily enters the alveoli from atmospheric air.

From alveoli into the blood

The partial pressure of oxygen in the pulmonary capillary is 40 mm Hg and in the alveoli it is 104 mm Hg. The pressure gradient of 64 mm Hg, facilitates the diffusion of oxygen from alveoli into the blood. The content of oxygen in arterial blood is 19 ml% and 14 ml% in venous blood. Thus, the diffusion of oxygen from alveoli to blood is 5 ml/100 ml of blood.

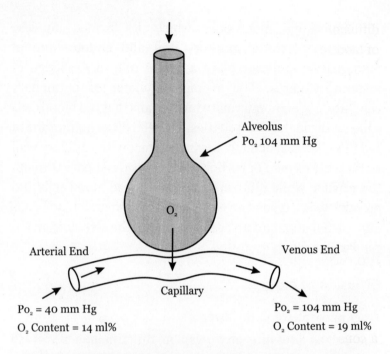

Fig.: 5.3 – Diffusion of oxygen from alveolus to pulmonary capillary

Diffusion of oxygen from blood into the tissues

The partial pressure of oxygen in arterial blood is 95 mm Hg. This is because of admixture of venous blood resulted by 2% of shunt flow i.e., 2% of blood reaches the heart without getting oxygenated. The average oxygen tension in the tissues is only 40 mm Hg. This is because of continuous metabolic activity and constant utilization of oxygen. Thus, a pressure gradient of about 55 mm Hg exists between blood and tissues so that, oxygen can easily diffuse into the tissues.

As mentioned above, the content of oxygen in arterial blood is 19 ml% and 14 ml% in venous blood. Thus, the diffusion of oxygen from blood to the tissues is 5 ml/100 ml of blood.

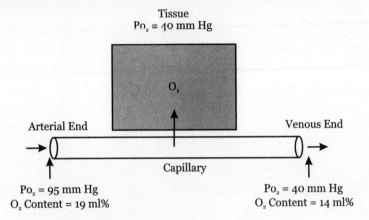

Fig.: 5.4 – Diffusion of oxygen from capillary to tissue

Approximately 250 ml of oxygen is used every minute by a conscious resting person and therefore about 25% of the arterial oxygen is used every minute.

Transport of oxygen: Oxygen is transported in blood in two forms,

1. As simple physical solution.

2. In combination with haemoglobin.

Oxygen dissolves in plasma and is transported in 0.3 ml/100 ml of plasma in physical form. In vertebrates, oxygen is diffused through membranes in the lungs and into the red blood cells.

As oxygen is one of the major substances required for chemical reactions in the cells, it is fortunate that the body has a special control mechanism to maintain an almost exact and constant oxygen concentration in the extracellular fluid. This mechanism depends principally on the chemical characteristics of haemoglobin, which is present in all red blood cells. Haemoglobin combines with oxygen as the blood passes through the lungs. Then, as the blood passes through the tissue capillaries, haemoglobin, does not release oxygen into the tissue fluid if too much oxygen is already there. But if the oxygen concentration in the tissue fluid is too low, sufficient oxygen is released to re-establish an adequate concentration. Thus, regulation of oxygen concentration in the tissues is vested principally in the chemical characteristics of haemoglobin itself. This regulation is called the oxygen-buffering function of haemoglobin.

Haemoglobin binds with oxygen and changes its colour from bluish red to bright red. Oxygen combines with haemoglobin in the blood and is transported as oxyhaemoglobin which is important because, as much as 97% of oxygen is transported by this method. In short, about 97% of the oxygen is transported from the lungs to the tissues is carried in chemical combination with haemoglobin in the red blood cells. The remaining 3% is transported in dissolved state in the water of plasma and blood cells. Thus, under normal conditions, oxygen is carried to the tissues almost entirely by haemoglobin.

One gram of haemoglobin carries 1.34 ml of oxygen called as oxygen carrying capacity of haemoglobin. The fetal haemoglobin has more affinity for oxygen than adult haemoglobin. Oxygen combines with haemoglobin only as a physical combination (by oxygenation). Thus, oxygen can be readily released from haemoglobin when it is needed. Haemoglobin accepts oxygen readily whenever the partial pressure of oxygen in the blood is more and gives out oxygen whenever the partial pressure of oxygen in the blood is less. Oxygen combines with the iron in heme part of haemoglobin. The oxygen carrying capacity of blood is 19 ml%. At low partial pressures of oxygen, most haemoglobin is deoxygenated. At around 90% oxygen saturation increases according to an oxygen-haemoglobin dissociation curve and approaches 100% at partial oxygen pressures greater than 10kPa. An arterial oxygen saturation value below 90% causes hypoxemia and indicated by cyanosis.

Venous oxygen saturation is measured to see how much oxygen the body consumes. Under clinical treatment, venous oxygen saturation below 60% indicates that the body is in lack of oxygen, and ischemic diseases occur.

Role of oxygen in respiratory control

In addition to control of respiratory activity by the respiratory center itself, still another mechanism is available for controlling respiration. This is the peripheral chemoreceptor system, shown in the following figure. Special nervous chemical receptors, called chemoreceptors, are located in several areas outside the brain. They are especially important for detecting changes in oxygen in the blood.

The chemoreceptors transmit nervous signals to the respiratory center in the brain to help regulate respiratory activity.

Most of the chemoreceptors are in the carotid bodies. However, a few are also in the aortic bodies, shown in the lower part of the following figure, and a very few are located elsewhere in association with other arteries of the thoracic and abdominal regions.

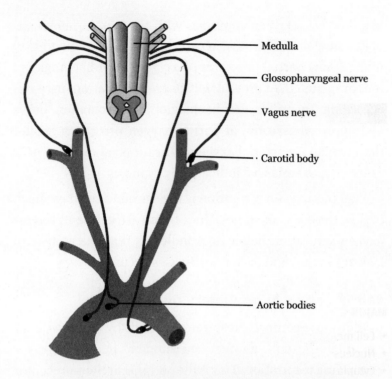

Fig.: 5.5 – Respiratory control by peripheral chemoreceptors in the carotid and aortic bodies

The carotid bodies are located bilaterally in the bifurcations of the common carotid arteries. Their afferent nerve fibers pass through Hering's nerves to the glossopharyngeal nerves and then to the dorsal respiratory area of the medulla. The aortic bodies are located along the arch of the aorta; their afferent nerve fibers pass through the vagi, also to the dorsal medullar respiratory area.

When the oxygen concentration in the arterial blood falls below normal, the chemoreceptors become strongly stimulated. This mechanism responds when the blood oxygen falls too low, mainly below a Po_2 of 70 mm Hg. This chapter thus gives the complete physiology of oxygen.

Cell and Oxygen Physiology

MAJOR CELL STRUCTURES AND ITS FUNCTIONS

- Cell membrane
- Nucleus
- Cytoplasm and organelles - cytoskeleton, ribosomes, endoplasmic reticulum, golgi apparatus or complex, lysosomes, centrioles and centrosomes, flagella and cilla
- Mitochondrion
  —Origin
  —Dysfunction and disease
  —Structure
  —Functions
  —Dysfunction and disease

NORMAL CELLULAR AGEING AND DEATH

- Cellular ageing
- Cell Death

CHAPTER 6

Cell and Oxygen Physiology

As we understand that vital force is nothing but oxygen energy, and is responsible for every cell's life. The inadequate consumption of oxygen in a cell causes disorders leading to dysfunction. In each and every cell nature has provided an excellent network for maintaining the proper balance between inspiration and expiration of gases. Also, it has its own metabolic unit to maintain adequate level of glucose, fat and protein. The production of aerobic energy takes place only in the presence of vital energy i.e. oxygen.

Cell is the basic structural and functional unit of the living body. The entire body contains about 100 trillion cells. Each organ is an aggregate of many different cells held together by intracellular supporting structures. Each type of cell is specially adapted to perform one or a few particular functions. In every cell the smallest amount of oxygen is stored for immediate use and for multiple intracellular activities. Without this oxygen energy, there will be immediate disturbance in cellular activities. Lack of oxygen is thus hazardous to every single cell.

So, let us try to understand in brief the cell structure and its functions.

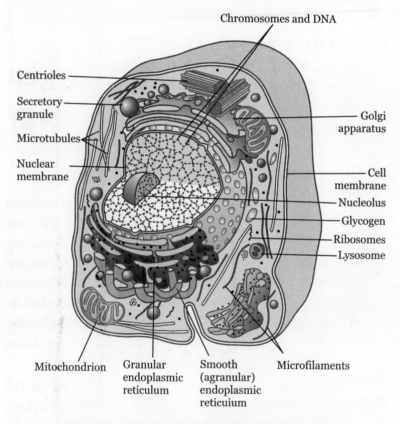

Fig.: 6.1 – A typical cell, showing the internal organelles in the cytoplasm and in the nucleus

MAJOR CELL STRUCTURES AND ITS FUNCTIONS

Each cell is formed by cell membrane, nucleus, and cytoplasm.

Cell membrane

It separates the cell body from the fluid surrounding the cell and serves as the boundary of the cell.

It is composed of three types of substances namely proteins 55%, lipids 40% and carbohydrates 5%.

Functions of cell membrane

1. Oxygen enters the cell from the blood and carbon dioxide leaves the cell and enters the blood through the cell membrane.
2. It protects the cytoplasm and the organelles of the cytoplasm.
3. The nutrients are absorbed into the cell through the cell membrane.
4. The metabolites and other waste products are excreted out through cell membrane.
5. Protein and carbohydrate molecules on the outer surface of cell membrane perform various functions; for example, they serve as markers that identify cells of each individual or as receptor molecules for certain hormones.

Nucleus

Dictates protein synthesis, thereby playing an essential role in other cell activities, namely active transport, metabolism, growth, and heredity.

Nucleus consists of:

1. An outer nuclear membrane studded with ribosomes and is continuous with endoplasmic reticulum.
2. Nuclear chromatin in the form of chromosomes which

are composed of three components DNA, RNA, and nuclear proteins.

3. Nucleolus: It consists of deoxyribonucleic acid (DNA), which programs the formation of RNA, and protein, which makes ribosomes.

Cytoplasm and organelles

It consists of:

1. **Cytoskeleton**–Includes three types of protein filaments (microfilaments, intermediate filaments, and microtubules) that give the cell shape and allow coordinated movements of organelles; in some cells the cytoskeleton is responsible for movement of the cell itself.

2. **Mitochondria**

3. **Ribosomes:** Are tiny granules that contain ribosomal RNA and many ribosomal proteins. Synthesise proteins; the 'Protein Factories' of the cell.

4. **Endoplasmic reticulum:** Membrane – bounded network of channels that provides surface area for many types of chemical reactions; ribosomes attached to rough endoplasmic reticulum synthesize proteins; smooth endoplasmic reticulum synthesizes lipids and certain carbohydrates.

5. **Golgi apparatus or complex:** Synthesizes carbohydrates, combines them with proteins, and packages the product as globules of glycoproteins.

6. **Lysosomes:** are membranous walled. It contains powerful lysosomal digestive (hydrolytic) enzymes, so are called as 'digestive system' of the cell.

7. **Centrioles and centrosomes:** are paired, rod shaped organelles. Each centriole is composed of microtubules that play an important role in the process of cell division. They also perform the function of formation and regeneration of cilia and flagella.

8. **Flagella and cilia:** allow movement of entire cell (flagella) or movement of substances along surface of cell (cilia).

Mitochondrion

Mitochondrion and oxygen are essential components for each other. Both depend on each other for their function. Mitochondria are workshop for oxygen.

From Homeopathic point of view, oxygen processed (development) in mitochondria is nothing but vital force.

Any disturbance in mitochondrion function will thus disturb the oxygen utility and hamper ATP production. This imbalance in group of cells proves to be the root cause of the disease.

Mitochondrion (plural mitochondria) is a membrane-enclosed organelle found in most eukaryotic cells. Mitochondria are rod shaped or oval shaped structure with a diameter of 0.5 – 1 micrometers (μm). Mitochondria are sometimes described as *'Cellular Power Plants'* because they generate most of the cell's supply of adenosine triphosphate (ATP). Without them, cells would be unable to extract enough energy from the nutrients, and essentially all cellular functions would cease.

Several characteristics make mitochondria unique. Mitochondria are present in all areas of each cell's cytoplasm, but the total number per cell varies from less than a hundred up to several thousand, depending on the amount of energy required by the cell. Further, the mitochondria are concentrated in those portions of the cell that are responsible for the major share of its energy metabolism. The mitochondrial proteome is thought to be dynamically regulated.

Origin

A mitochondrion contains DNA, which is organized as several copies of a single, circular chromosome.

Mitochondrial genome is a circular DNA molecule. One mitochondrion can contain two to ten copies of its DNA.

Mitochondria are self-replicative, which means that one mitochondrion can form a second one, a third one, and so on, whenever there is a need in the cell for increased amounts of ATP. Indeed, the mitochondria contain DNA similar to that found in the cell nucleus. The DNA of the mitochondrion plays a similar role, controlling replication of the mitochondrion itself.

Structure

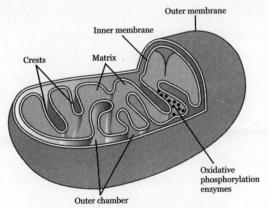

Fig.: 6.2 – Structure of a Mitochondrion

The basic structure of the mitochondrion is composed mainly of two lipid bilayer-protein membranes: an outer membrane and an inner membrane. Many infoldings of the inner membrane form shelves onto which oxidative enzymes are attached. In addition, the inner cavity of the mitochondrion is filled with a matrix that contains large quantities of dissolved enzymes that are necessary for extracting energy from nutrients.

The matrix is important in the production of ATP with the aid of the ATP synthase contained in the inner membrane. Mitochondria have their own genetic material, and the machinery to manufacture their own RNAs and proteins.

Functions

1. Energy Conversion

   The most prominent roles of the mitochondrion are its production of ATP and regulation of cellular metabolism. This is done by oxidizing the major products of glucose, pyruvate, and NADH, which are produced in the cytosol, obtained from the catabolism of digested food particles - proteins, carbohydrates and lipids. This process of cellular respiration, also known as aerobic respiration, is dependent on the presence of oxygen.

   The energy produced in mitochondria is stored in the form of chemical energy bound to the adenosine triphosphate (ATP) molecules.

   Whenever, there is need for energy, the ATP molecules are broken and there is release of energy. Mitochondria contain many enzymes responsible for Krebs cycle, oxidative phosphorylation and synthesis of ATP.

   • Pyruvate: The Citric Acid Cycle

Each pyruvate molecule produced by glycolysis is actively transported across the inner mitochondrial membrane, and into the matrix where it is oxidized and combined with coenzyme A to form CO_2, acetyl-CoA, and NADH.

- NADH and $FADH_2$: The Electron Transport Chain

The redox energy from NADH and $FADH_2$ is transferred to oxygen (O_2) in several steps via the electron transport chain. These energy-rich molecules are produced within the matrix via the citric acid cycle but are also produced in the cytoplasm by glycolysis. Protein complexes in the inner membrane (NADH dehydrogenase, cytochrome c reductase and cytochrome c oxidase perform the transfer and the incremental release of energy is used to pump protons (H+) into the intermembrane space. As the proton concentration increases in the intermembrane space, a strong electrochemical gradient is established across the inner membrane. The protons can return to the matrix through the ATP synthase complex, and their potential energy is used to synthesize ATP from ADP and inorganic phosphate (Pi). This process is called chemiosmosis. This process is efficient, but a small percentage of electrons may prematurely reduce oxygen, forming reactive oxygen species such as superoxide. This can cause oxidative stress in the mitochondria and may contribute to the decline in mitochondrial function associated with the aging process.

2. Heat production
3. Storage of calcium ions

Mitochondria can transiently store calcium, a contributing process for the cell's homeostasis of calcium. In fact, their ability to rapidly take in calcium for later release makes them very good 'Cytosolic Buffers' for calcium. Release of calcium back into the cell's interior can initiate calcium spikes or calcium waves with large changes in the membrane potential. These can activate a series of second messenger system proteins that can coordinate processes such as neurotransmitter release in nerve cells and release of hormones in endocrine cells.

4. Regulation of the membrane potential

5. Apoptosis-programmed cell death

6. Calcium signaling (including calcium-evoked apoptosis)

7. Cellular proliferation regulation

8. Regulation of cellular metabolism

9. Certain haem synthesis reactions

10. Steroid synthesis

Some mitochondrial functions are performed only in specific types of cells. For example, mitochondria in liver cells contain enzymes that allow them to detoxify ammonia, a waste product of protein metabolism. A mutation in the genes regulating any of these functions can result in mitochondrial diseases.

Dysfunction and disease

With their central place in cell metabolism, damage and subsequent dysfunction in mitochondria is an important factor for all sorts of human diseases.

Disturbance of oxidative phosphorylation is central to mitochondrial disease. Many other factors such as dishomeostasis increased oxidative stress and defective turnover of mitochondrial protein also contribute. Likewise, the cell dysfunctioning and diseases occur.

NORMAL CELLULAR AGEING AND DEATH

Cellular ageing and death are common physiological processes. They are natural functions of the cell cycle.

Cellular ageing

As the cell ages, it becomes less efficient in carrying out its functions. It also is more at risk of damage from harmful environmental agents. With progressive damage, cells lose their ability to repair themselves. In time, they begin to malfunction. Examples of the manifestations of ageing cells include gray hair, reduced muscle mass, menopause, arteriosclerosis, memory and vision impairment, and arthritis.

Ageing is caused by progressive and reversible molecular oxidative damage due to persistent oxidative stress on the human cells. In normal cells, very small amount (3%) of total oxygen consumption by the cell is converted into reactive oxygen species. The rate of generation of reactive oxygen species is directly correlated with metabolic rate of the organisms. More the animal lowers the metabolic rate, longer will be his life span. The underlying mechanism appears to be oxidative damage to mitochondria with high mutation rates of mitochondrial DNA. A vicious cycle is thought to occur, as oxidative stress leads to mitochondrial DNA mutations, which can lead to enzymatic abnormalities and further oxidative stress. A number of changes occur to mitochondria during the aging process.

Cell Death

A cell dies if it has been irreparably damaged. Shortly after cell death, structural changes begin to occur in the nucleus and cytoplasm. The lysosome begins to undergo membrane breakdown. This releases the lysosomal enzymes, which begin to digest the cell. The nucleus shrinks and dissolves or breaks into fragments.

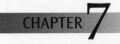
Role of Oxygen (Vital Energy) in Metabolism

CHAPTER 7

Role of Oxygen (Vital Energy) in Metabolism

Although many cells of the body often differ markedly from one another, all of them have certain basic characteristics that are alike. For instance, in all cells, oxygen reacts with carbohydrate, fat, and protein to release the energy required for cell function. Further, the general chemical mechanisms for converting nutrients into energy are basically the same in all cells, and all cells deliver end products of their chemical reactions into the surrounding fluids.

Oxygen energy takes part in the metabolic activity of each and every cell of living organism. Without oxidation there would be no energy creation and no functional activities in the organism. Every smallest organism absorbs oxygen energy through respiration and life begins from respiratory activity (inspiration and expiration) of the organism. Oxygen plays an important role in every moment of life.

In this chapter, the explanation about oxygen related cellular metabolism of carbohydrates, fats, and proteins is given in short. (Only catabolism that is energy generating process is explained.)

The principle substances from which cells extract energy are foodstuffs that react chemically with oxygen-viz carbohydrates, fats, and proteins. In the human body, essentially all carbohydrates are converted into glucose by the digestive tract and liver before they reach the other cells of the body. Similarly, proteins are converted into amino acids, and fats into fatty acids. Oxygen and foodstuffs – glucose, fatty acids, and amino acids – all enter the cell. Inside the cell, the foodstuffs react chemically with oxygen, under the influence of enzymes that control the reactions and channel the energy released in the proper direction.

PHOSPHORYLATION

Phosphorylation includes all chemical reactions in the body which require combination with phosphoric acid.

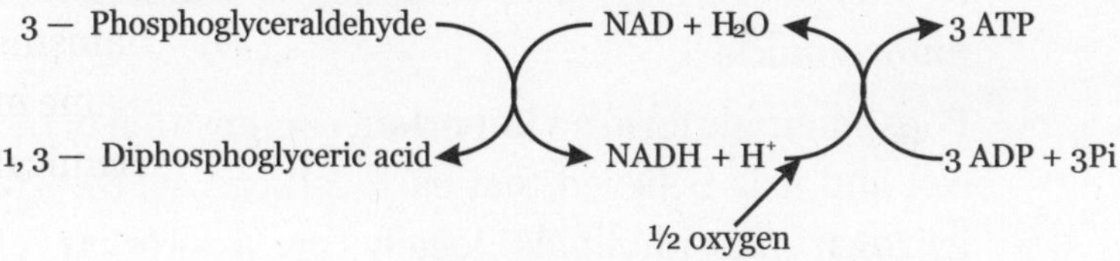

3 — Phosphoglyceraldehyde ⟶ NAD + H_2O ⟵ ⟶ 3 ATP

1, 3 — Diphosphoglyceric acid ⟵ ⟶ NADH + H^+ — 3 ADP + 3Pi

½ oxygen

[Through Electron Transport Chain]

Fig.: 7.1 – Schematic representation of oxidative phosphorylation

Phosphoric acid enters into the composition of cell protoplasm. Phosphorylation is an important chemical process for all cells. In addition to this, it takes an essential part during absorption and metabolism of different foodstuffs. Its effect in the different channels of metabolism are as follows:

1. In relation to carbohydrates: Absorption of carbohydrates through the intestinal mucosa and also re-absorption of glucose from renal tubules, are helped by oxidative phosphorylation.

   • Formation of glycogen from glucose and breakdown of glycogen into glucose in the liver and muscles takes place through phosphorylation.

   • During chemical changes accompanying muscular contraction, phosphorylation takes place at all important steps.

2. In relation to fats: During absorption of fats, neutral fats and phospholipids are synthesized in the absorbing epithelium. Phosphorylation is carried out by the enzyme phosphorylase.

   • Liver synthesizes phospholipids, especially lecithin. It is a very important step in the transport of fat. It also acts as a primary stage in the further oxidation of fatty acids. Fatty acid oxidation is a function of mitochondria.

   • Phospholipids form an important composition of the cell and it is believed that each cell can synthesize its own phospholipids locally by a process of phosphorylation.

3. In relation to proteins: It is an important step by which all the phosphoproteins are synthesized, such as, nucleoproteins, caseinogens, etc.

   Phosphorylation takes an important part in tissue oxidation during which proteins, fats and carbohydrates are finally broken down.

4. Formation of bone is another example of phosphorylation.

KREBS CYCLE OR CITRIC ACID CYCLE

The Krebs cycle is one of the most important biochemical mechanisms of oxidation of the activated metabolites and it is perhaps the major terminal pathway of biological oxidation in all animal tissues. The activated metabolites, which are few in number derived from carbohydrate, protein, and fat are oxidized by the electron-transport chain and most of the utilizable energy is produced for the organism.

This cycle includes series of oxidation-reduction reactions in which coenzymes (NAD^+ and FAD) pick up hydrogen ions and hydride ions from oxidized organic acids, and some ATP is produced. CO_2 and H_2O are the by-products.

Carbohydrate Metabolism

Complete oxidation of glucose, also referred to as cellular respiration, is the chief source of ATP in cells. The process requires glycolysis, Krebs cycle, and electron transport chain. The complete oxidation of 1 molecule of glucose yields a maximum of 38 molecules of ATP. The process of breakdown of glycogen to glucose and further to pyruvic acid is anaerobic.

This pyruvic acid is converted into acetyl Coenzyme-A with release of 4 hydrogen atoms and then it enters in Krebs cycle and further oxidized to carbon dioxide and water.

Third set of reactions in glucose catabolism is another series of oxidation – reduction reactions, in which electrons are passed from one carrier to the next, and most of the ATP is produced and these reactions requires oxygen.

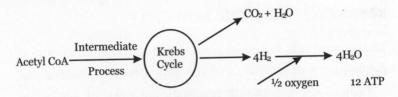

Fig. 7.2: Carbohydrate Metabolism

Fat metabolism

Triglycerides are broken down into glycerol and fatty acids. Glycerol may be converted into glucose (gluconeogenesis) or catabolised via glycolysis. Fatty acid oxidation takes place in a process known as alternate successive beta-oxidation. Consequently, the original fatty acid molecule is converted into several molecules of acetic acid and one molecule of acetoacetic acid. Both of these compounds undergo final oxidation into carbon dioxide and water in Krebs cycle.

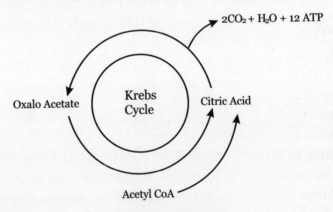

Fig. 7.3: Fat Metabolism

Protein Metabolism

The metabolism of protein is meant by metabolism of amino acids. Amino acids are oxidized via the Krebs cycle after deamination. Ammonia resulting from deamination is converted into urea in the liver, passed into blood, and excreted in urine. Amino acids may be converted into glucose (gluconeogenesis), fatty acids, or ketone bodies.

When, only carbohydrate is utilized, one molecule of carbon dioxide is formed for every molecule of oxygen consumed.

When fat is utilized, oxygen reacts with fats and a large portion of oxygen combines with hydrogen ions to form water instead of carbon dioxide. Because of this, carbon dioxide output is less.

Briefly, almost all these oxidative reactions occur inside the mitochondria, and the energy that is released is used to form the high – energy compound ATP. Then, ATP, not the original foodstuffs, is used throughout the cell to energize almost all the subsequent intracellular metabolic reactions.

Effect of intracellular Po_2 on rate of oxygen usage

Only a minute level of oxygen pressure is required in the cells for normal intracellular chemical reactions to take place. The reason for this is that the respiratory enzyme systems of the cell are geared so that when the cellular Po_2 is more than 1 mm Hg, oxygen availability is no longer a limiting factor in the rates of the chemical reactions. Instead, the main limiting factor is the concentration of adenosine diphosphate (ADP) in the cells. Whenever the intracellular Po_2 is above 1 mm Hg, the rate of oxygen usage becomes constant for any given concentration of ADP in the cell. Conversely, when the ADP concentration is alterd, the rate of oxygen usage changes in proportion to the change in ADP concentration. Under normal operating conditions, the rate of oxygen usage by the cells is controlled ultimately by the rate of energy expenditure within the cells – that is, by the rate at which ADP is formed from ATP.

Effect of blood flow on metabolic use of oxygen

The total amount of oxygen available each minute for use in any given tissue is determined by

1. The quantity of oxygen that can be transported to the tissue in each 100 milliliters of blood and

2. The rate of blood flow.

If the rate of blood flow falls to zero, the amount of available oxygen also falls to zero. Thus, there are times when the rate of blood flow through a tissue can be so low that tissue Po_2 falls below the critical 1 mm Hg required for intracellular metabolism. Under these conditions, the rate of tissue usage of oxygen is blood flow limited. Neither diffusion-limited nor blood flow-limited oxygen states can continue for long, because the cells receive less oxygen than is required to continue the life of the cells.

Adenosine triphosphate (ATP)

It is a multifunctional nucleotide and plays an important role in cell biology as a co-enzyme that is the molecular unit of currency, of intracellular energy transfer. In this role, ATP transports chemical energy within cells for metabolism. It is produced as an energy source during the processes of cellular respiration, biosynthetic reactions, motility, and cell division.

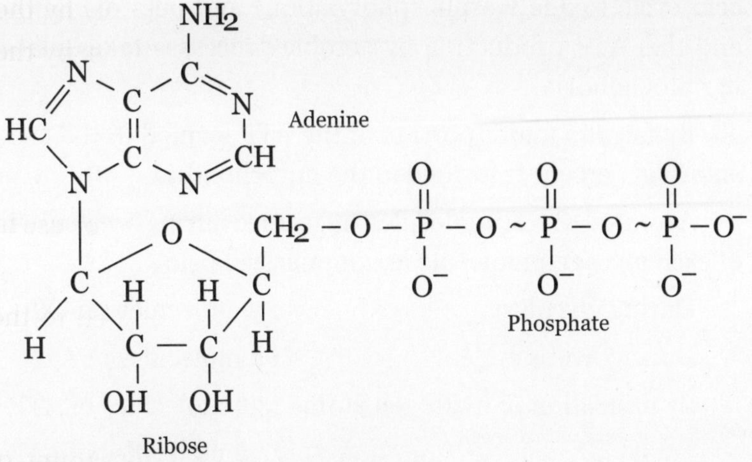

Fig. 7.4: Diagrammatic molecular formula of Adenosine Triphosphate

ATP is a nucleotide composed of:

1. The nitrogenous base adenine

2. The pentose sugar ribose

3. Three phosphate radicals

ATP is present everywhere in the cytoplasm and nucleoplasm of all cells, and essentially all the physiologic mechanisms that require energy for operation obtain it directly from ATP. In turn, the food in the cells is gradually oxidized, and the released energy is used to form new ATP, thus always maintaining a supply of this substance. All these energy transfers take place by means of coupled reactions.

Apart from the important role being played by it in energy metabolism and signaling, ATP is also incorporated into nucleic acids by polymerases in process of DNA replication and transcription.

ATP can be produced by a number of distinct cellular processes. The three main pathways used are glycolysis, citric acid cycle (oxidative phosphorylation) and beta oxidation and this ATP production by aerobic processes takes place in mitochondria.

By far, the major portion of the ATP formed in the cell, about 95 percent is formed in the mitochondria.

A total of 38 ATP molecules are formed during breakdown of each glycogen molecule as summarized below.

During glycolysis : 2 molecules of ATP

During Krebs cycle : 2 molecules of ATP

By utilization of hydrogen atoms : 34 molecules of ATP

Total : 38 molecules of ATP

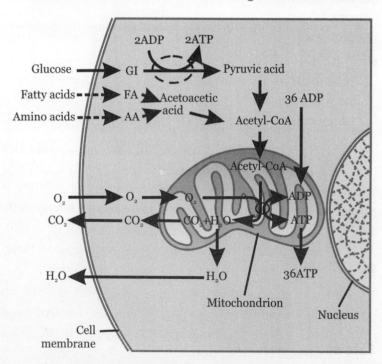

Fig. 7.5: Formation of ATP in the cell, showing that most of the ATP is formed in the mitochondria

Functions of ATP in cells

1. Synthesis of macromolecules, including DNA, RNA, and proteins.

2. Transport of macromolecules across cell membranes.

3. ATP is critically involved in maintaining cell structure by facilitating assemble and disassembly of elements of cytoskeleton.

4. ATP is required for the shortening of actin and myosin filament cross bridges for muscle contraction and performance of mechanical work.

5. Cell signaling: ATP is also a signaling molecule. This signaling role is important in both the lateral and peripheral nervous system.

6. Intracellular signaling: ATP is critical in signal transduction processes. Kinase activity on substrate such as proteins or membrane lipids is common form of signal transduction. Through cyclic AMP it triggers calcium signals by release of Calcium from intracellular stores. This form of signaling is important in brain function and multitude of other cellular processes.

7. It is required for various synthetic reactions that create hormones, cell membranes, and many other essential molecules of the body.

8. Cell division and growth.

9. Many other physiologic functions those are necessary to maintain and propagate life.

Fate of Anaerobic Metabolism

In the healthy body, most cellular metabolism is aerobic metabolism. Occasionally oxygen becomes unavailable or insufficient so that oxidative phosphorylation cannot take place and anaerobic metabolism results. Even under these conditions, small amount of energy can be released by the glycolysis stage of carbohydrate degradation. It generates 2 ATP molecules for every molecule of glucose whereas aerobic metabolism generates 36 ATP molecules for every molecule of glucose. This anaerobic process is extremely wasteful of glucose because only 24,000 cal. of energy are used to form ATP for each molecule of glucose metabolized which represents only a little over 3 percent of total energy in the glucose molecules. This release of glycolytic energy to the cells called as anaerobic energy which is only useful for few minutes when oxygen is unavailable and it can supply only a small fraction of the energy.

By itself, anaerobic metabolism cannot meet the body's energy needs and with anaerobic metabolism, the rate of glycolysis must be greatly increased to meet the body's energy demands. This leads to an increase in the production of lactic acid and resultant metabolic acidosis. As tissue metabolites (and hydrogen ions) continue to accumulate, they stimulate vasodilatation. This vasodilatation opposes the hormonally regulated constriction of the pre-capillary sphincters, thereby reducing the body's ability to continue vital tissue perfusion by maintaining the proper size of the vascular compartment. This in turn, increases the capillary hydrostatic pressure. The result is fluid loss from the vascular space into the interstitial space. In addition, the insufficient energy production of anaerobic metabolism affects the cells' ability to maintain normal sodium – potassium differential across the cell membrane. Intracellular potassium leaks out of the cell; sodium leaks into the cell. This creates cellular swelling and a decreased transmembrane potential. Energy production is further impaired. Finally, the cells are irreversibly damaged.

Thus, at the end of this chapter, we come to the conclusion that oxygen is essential for metabolic activities and the energy creating activities. Energy is required for all of the cellular activities that support life.

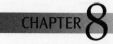
Exercise and Oxygen

CLASSIFICATION OF EXERCISE

- Severe exercise/violent exercise
- Moderate exercise
- Mild exercise/non-violent exercise

FACTORS INVOLVED IN INCREASING THE PULMONARY VENTILATION DURING EXERCISE

CHAPTER 8

Exercise and Oxygen

Healthy functioning of cell requires uninterrupted supply of oxygen for production of ATP and lack of oxygen creates illness in the body.

Increased requirement of energy during exercise calls for increase in demand of oxygen (vital force) for the purpose of energy creation.

Exercise increase intake of oxygen (vital force) by the body and thereby facilitates to maintain healthy state. Thus, exercise not only keeps the body healthy but also helps healing the diseased or injured cells due to good oxygen supply.

Muscular exercise brings about a lot of changes on various systems of the body. The degree of changes depends upon the severity of exercise. Thus, accordingly exercise is classified as:

1. **Severe exercise / Violent exercise:** It involves strenuous muscular activity. Complete exhaustion occurs at the end of severe exercise. For example, fast running, for a distance of 100 or 400 meters.

2. **Moderate exercise:** This does not involve strenuous muscular activity. So, this type of exercise can be performed for a longer period and exhaustion does not occur at the end of moderate exercise. For example, fast walking.

3. **Mild exercise / Non-violent exercise:** It is useful even in the diseased or ill state to enhance the oxygen flow in the body. Example: Yoga-asana, pranayam or breathing exercise, stretching exercise.

During exercise, the muscles need more oxygen and various respiratory and cardiovascular adjustments take place to cope with increased need for oxygen. All the adjustments are aimed at increasing the pulmonary ventilation, diffusing capacity for oxygen and supply of more amount of oxygen to muscles so that, the muscles can consume more oxygen. During exercise, hyperventilation occurs which includes increase in rate and force of respiration. For example, in moderate exercise, respiratory rate is about 30/min, tidal volume increases to about 2000 ml and pulmonary ventilation is about 60 litres/min.

Factors involved in increasing the pulmonary ventilation during exercise:

1. Activation of higher centers accelerates the respiratory processes by stimulating respiratory centres.

2. The chemoreceptors send impulses to the respiratory centres, which in turn increase the rate and force of respiration.

3. The proprioceptors are activated very much; send impulses to brain particularly, the cerebral cortex through somatic afferent nerves. Cerebral cortex in turn

causes hyperventilation by stimulating the medullary respiratory centres.

4. Increased body temperature and acidosis during exercise enhance the ventilation by stimulating respiratory centres.

The oxygen consumed by the tissues, particularly the skeletal muscles is greatly enhanced during exercise. The cause is vasodilatation in muscles, increase in blood flow, and more amount of oxygen diffusing from blood into the muscles. After a period of severe muscular exercise, the amount of oxygen consumed is enormously more. The oxygen required is more than the quantity available to the muscle. This much of oxygen is utilized for the reversal of the following metabolic processes.

1. Reformation of glucose from lactic acid accumulated during exercise.

2. Re-synthesis of ATP and creatine phosphate.

3. Restoration of amount of oxygen dissociated from haemoglobin and myoglobin.

During exercise, blood flow through the pulmonary capillaries is increased. Because of this the diffusing capacity of alveoli for oxygen is increased. The mild hypoxia developed during exercise stimulates the juxtaglomerular apparatus to secrete erythropoietin. This stimulates the bone marrow and causes release of red blood cells.

At the onset of exercise, signals are transmitted not only from the brain to the muscles to cause muscle contraction but also into the vasomotor center to initiate mass sympathetic discharge throughout the body. Simultaneously, the parasympathetic signals to the heart are attenuated.

Cardiac output is increased up to 20 litres/min in moderate exercise and up to 35 litres/min during severe exercise. The increase in cardiac output is directly proportional to the increase in the amount of oxygen consumed during exercise.

Here, we can understand how demand and supply ratio changes during slow and rapid physical activities like exercise. Oxygen demand increases along with the release of energy. The different types of body receptors give the immediate response and signal to our central nervous system to accelerate the breathing rate and thus maintains homeostasis of internal environment of the body.

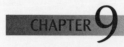
CHAPTER 9

How Symptoms Manifest in Human Body?

SYMPTOMS

SENSATION

DISEASE

ISCHAEMIA – CAUSE OF PAIN

How Symptoms Manifest in Human Body?

When the body is in equilibrium, the functions and the sensations in the body and mind are in normally active and balanced state. This is the state where the human being feels contentment. The body feels at ease, weightless, trouble-free along with complete physical, mental, & social harmony.

Usually, if any changes occur in the body or its function, it is perceived by the patient. **Symptoms** represent subjective experience of the disease, which is narrated by the patient in their complaints or history of present illness.

The various aspects of general symptom analysis includes mode of onset, progress (gradual or sudden), duration and precipitating factors, characteristics, location, radiation, severity, timing aggravation [<] & amelioration [>] factors.

These symptoms are expressed by various kinds of abnormal sensations. **Sensation** means a feeling or awareness of the conditions within the body resulting from the stimulation of sensory receptors.

The word **'disease'** is produced by mixture of two words

i.e. dis + ease. The man, who is not at ease, is in disease. The concept of disease and illness differs in that disease is usually measurable whereas illness is highly individual and personal. Thus, a person may have a serious but symptom free disease i.e. hypertension, diabetes mellitus and even myocardial infarction.

As from the homeopathic point of view, when we are treating the sick i.e. the unwell-being of the person, the homeopathic physician must consider the physical generals and characteristic symptoms along with mental symptoms (i.e. patient as a whole).

Usually the symptoms and the abnormal sensations indicate that there is some dysfunction in the human body. Whenever there is less oxygen supply, at that time the cells start their abnormal behavior and at the same time changes occur in aerobic metabolism. The indication of this abnormal behavior of the cell is received by the different receptors and they give information through the nerves to the brain. So the lack of oxygen is most probably responsible for all kinds of symptoms.

Whenever the body is in well being state, each and every cell receives appropriate amount of oxygen via the respiratory system. Lack of oxygen leads to cell injury which depends on the duration of hypoxia and every physician make an effort to find out the cause for the oxygen lack in human body.

Disease occurs due to lack of ease in the cellular metabolic process. Multiple biochemical disturbances occur in metabolic pathway leading to various diseases; for example - atherosclerosis, diabetes mellitus, hyperlipidemia etc. for which again disturbance in oxygen energy or vital force is responsible. The symptoms, abnormal sensations, and dysfunction in the body occur due to inappropriate oxygen supply. Example, pain occurs whenever any tissues are being damaged, and it causes the individual to react to remove the pain stimulus. Even such simple activities as sitting for a long time on the ischia can cause tissue destruction because of lack of blood flow to the skin where it is compressed by the weight of the body. When skin becomes painful as a result of the ischaemia, the person normally shifts body weight subconsciously.

When blood flow to a tissue is blocked, (ischaemia) the tissue often becomes very painful within a few minutes. The greater the rate of metabolism of the tissue, the more rapidly the pain appears. One of the suggested causes of pain during ischaemia is accumulation of large amounts of lactic acid in the tissues formed as a consequence of anaerobic metabolism. Probably, other chemical agents, such as bradykinin and proteolytic enzymes, are formed in the tissues because of cell damage and these stimulate the pain nerve endings.

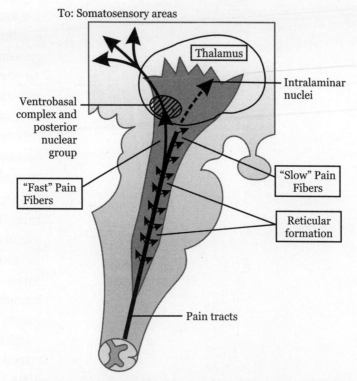

Fig. 9.1: Transmission of pain signals into the brain stem, thalamus, and cerebral cortex by way of the fast pricking pain pathway and the slow burning pain pathway

The physiology behind the pain is ischemic condition of the affected tissue which releases the pain stimulation through the receptor to the neuron and message is sent through hypothalamus and cerebral cortex. It indicates alarming situation to the body and the central nervous system takes appropriate decision according to pain stimulation. Here, again it is important indication that pain is a manifestation of lack of oxygen (vital force) to the body.

Relation of Oxygen to Disease State

FREE RADICALS-MEDIATED CELL INJURY

CAUSES OF CELL INJURY

- Hypoxia and ischaemia
  - —Reversible cell injury
  - —Irreversible cell injury
- The most important cause of vital energy derangement: hypoxia
  - —Types of hypoxia
  - —Local effects of hypoxia
  - —Effect of hypoxia on synaptic transmission
  - —The relation of vital force with hypoxia
  - — Effects of foetal hypoxia
- Physical & chemical injuries
  - —Physical injuries
  - —Chemical injuries
- Microbial agents
  - —Bacteria
  - —Viruses
  - —Fungi
  - —Parasites
- Immunologic agents
- Nutritional derangements
- Genetic factors
- Psychological factor

CHAPTER 10

Relation of Oxygen to Disease State

In health, all expressions of vital force may be expressed by perfect functioning of all parts of the body and by a sense of general well-being.

In disease, this expression is vastly changed. There is a sense of discomfort. The mental expressions are vastly altered according to the degree of disturbance. The signs and symptoms appear and all because of the disturbed vital functions, either from external impressions having a depressing effect, and the consequent reaction of the vital force or from some hidden miasm coming into its full expression in its impression on the vital force. Thus, disease is a disturbed vital process.

Because of the impacts of these external impressions and the miasms, each and every cell of our body undergoes severe stress. This stressful situation affects the functioning of whole body and its microcellular organelles. Every disease is born through this process.

Most of the disease states begin with cell injury and consequent loss of cellular function. Cell injury is defined as a variety of stress a cell encounters as a result of changes in its internal and external environment.

In this chapter, I would like to specify the relation between the disturbed oxygen energy (vital energy) and disease process at the cellular level (cell organelle especially mitochondria).

Cells need an adequate and constant supply of oxygen. Without this, they cannot generate enough amount of energy to maintain the metabolism and mechanisms (example, ion pumps) that move some of the essential substances across the cell membrane.

Initially lack of oxygen affects the cellular function temporarily but with time irreversible damage is done and revitalization is impossible. Absence of vital force for just few minutes in the body creates a great hazard in each and every cell of living organism and obviously the result will be hypoxia, instant cell injury, and death. The cell cannot survive without this vital energy i.e. oxygen.

Free radicals-mediated cell injury

Within every cell there are small micro organelle called mitochondria. It is a power house of every cell which reduces oxygen by the transfer of electrons to create energy in the form of ATP and also produces a byproduct of water. This process goes without any hitch at least 90 to 98 percent. Generation of oxygen radicals begins within mitochondrial inner membrane when cytochrome oxidase catalyses the four electron reduction of oxygen (O_2) to water (H_2O). Intermediate between reactions of oxygen to water, three partially reduced species of oxygen are generated depending upon the number of electrons transferred. These are:

1. Superoxide oxygen (O'$_2$): one electron
2. Hydrogen peroxide (H$_2$O$_2$): two electrons
3. Hydroxyl radical (OH⁻): three electrons

Free radicals are electrically charged molecules that have an unpaired electron. Such molecules are unstable and highly reactive. When an oxygen free radical takes an electron from one molecule, that molecule becomes unstable and borrows an electron from another molecule, which, in turn, becomes unstable. These chain reactions lead to cellular damage and death. Among the molecules attacked by oxygen free radicals are proteins (such as enzymes), neurotransmitters, nucleic acid, and phospholipids of plasma membranes.

These free radicals are responsible for most of the life threatening diseases in our life. Whichever part of body receives the most free radicals damage, are the first to wear out and this results in degenerative diseases. If this process is developed in eyes, it causes macular degeneration or cataract and glaucoma type of diseases. In a blood vessel atherosclerosis develops which is responsible for infarction, in joints it leads to arthritis, in brain it causes Alzheimer's or Parkinson's disease, and in kidneys or liver the physiological function of that organ undergo damage and pathology develops.

When oxygen molecules maintain their strength there is energy and life, but the breakdown of oxygen create hazards in the life through the free radicals and this is called **oxidative stress.** This oxidative stress is underlying cause of almost all degenerative diseases. The aging process itself is an oxidative stress that is caused due to free radicals. The free radicals set off a chain reaction leading to potentially degenerative condition. Chemically the violent action of these free radicals has been shown to actually produce hazardous effect. Day to day breakdown of oxygen causes vital battle inside the body.

Free radicals-mediated cell injury plays an important role in the following situations:

1. Ischemic reperfusion injury
2. Ionizing radiation by causing radiolysis of water
3. Chemical toxicity
4. Hyperoxia (toxicity due to oxygen therapy)
5. Cellular aging
6. Killing of exogenous biologic agents
7. Inflammatory damage
8. Destruction of tumor cells
9. Chemical carcinogenesis
10. Atherosclerosis

Causes of cell injury

Every kind of cell injury creates some amounts of dysfunction in the mitochondria causing altered oxygen supply to the injured cell. The vital derangement initiated at this moment disturbs the cellular homeostasis. Let's see the various causes of vital derangement.

1. Hypoxia and Ischaemia
2. Physical & Chemical injuries
3. Microbial agents
4. Immunologic agents
5. Nutritional derangements

6. Genetic factors

7. Psychological factors

Hypoxia and Ischaemia

The interruption of the blood supply (ischaemia) and impaired oxygen supply to the tissues (hypoxia) are the most common form of cell injury in human beings. It causes reversible and irreversible cell injury.

Reversible cell injury

In reversible cell injury the sequential intracellular changes are as follows:

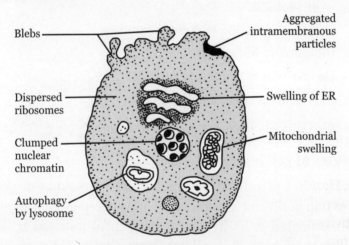

Blebs

Aggregated intramembranous particles

Dispersed ribosomes

Swelling of ER

Clumped nuclear chromatin

Mitochondrial swelling

Autophagy by lysosome

Fig. 10.1: Reversible cell injury

Decreased cellular ATP:

ATP is derived from two sources- firstly, by aerobic respiration in the mitochondria, and secondly, by anaerobic glycolytic pathway. Hypoxia and ischaemia both limit the supply of oxygen to the cells, thus causing decreased ATP generation.

Highly specialized cells as myocardium, proximal tubular

cells of the kidney and neurons of the central nervous system are dependent on aerobic ATP generation and thus suffer from ill-effects of ischaemia more severely and rapidly.

Decrease in intracellular pH:

Low oxygen supply to cell

↓

Failure of aerobic respiration by mitochondria

↓ followed by

Anaerobic glycolytic pathway for the energy (ATP) requirement.

↓ resulting in

Rapid depletion of glycogen and accumulation of lactic acid

↓ lowering

The intracellular pH

Fig. 10.2: Sequence leading to decreased intra-cellular pH due to lack of oxygen supply

Damage to plasma membrane sodium pump: Lowered ATP in the cell and consequent increased ATPase activity interfere with energy (ATP) dependant sodium pump. This results in intracellular accumulation of sodium and diffusion of potassium out of cell. This causes hydropic swelling that is increase in intracellular water to maintain iso-osmotic conditions

Reduced protein synthesis: As a result of continued hypoxia, ribosomes are detached from granular endoplasmic reticulum and polysomes are degraded to monosomes, thus causing decreased protein synthesis.

Functional consequences: Reversible cell injury may result in functional disturbances for eg. myocardial contractility ceases within 60 seconds of coronary occlusion but can be reversed if circulation is restored.

Ultrastructural changes: Following ultrastructural changes are seen in reversible cell injury:

1. Endoplasmic reticulum – Distension of cisternae by fluid and detachment of membrane bound polyribosome from the surface of rough endoplasmic reticulum.

2. Mitochondrial swelling and phospholipid rich amorphous densities.

3. Plasma membrane – Loss of microvilli and focal cytoplasmic projections.

4. Nucleolus – There is segregation of granular and febrile components of nucleolus and reduced synthesis of ribosomal RNA.

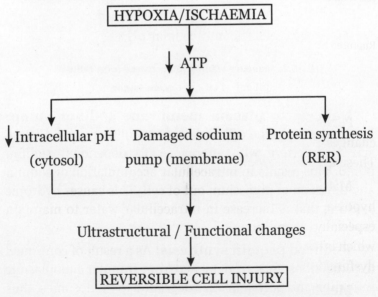

Fig. 10.3: Sequence of events in the pathogenesis of reversible cell injury caused by hypoxia / ischaemia

Irreversible cell injury

Two essential phenomena always distinguish irreversible from reversible cell injury.

1. Inability of the cell to reverse mitochondrial dysfunction on reperfusion or re-oxygenation.
2. Disturbance in cell membrane function in general.

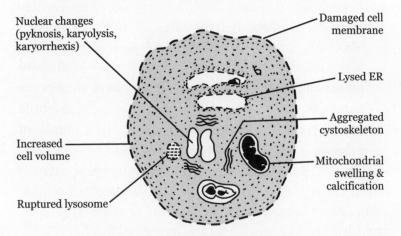

Fig. 10.4: Irreversible cell injury

Persistent hypoxia or ischaemia results in irreversible changes in structure and function of the cell (cell death). These are as follows:

Mitochondrial dysfunction: Due to continued hypoxia, a large cytosolic influx of calcium ions occurs, especially after reperfusion of irreversibly injured cell, which is taken up by mitochondria and causes mitochondrial dysfunction.

Membrane damage: Defect in membrane function, especially plasma membrane, is the most important event in irreversible cell injury in ischaemia. The mechanisms are:

1. Accelerated degradation of membrane phospholipid.

2. Damage to intermediate filaments of the cytoskeleton.

3. Toxic oxygen radicals. Reactive oxygen-derived species – superoxide, hydrogen peroxide, and hydroxyl radicals are increased in ischaemia.

4. Breakdown products of lipid.

5. Reperfusion damage – Upon reperfusion of irreversibly injured cell, there is large cytosolic influx of calcium ions. An increased cytosolic calcium concentration may activate membrane phospholipase leading to phospholipid degradation, to bring about membrane damage.

Hydrolytic enzymes: Damage to lysosomal membranes is followed by liberation of hydrolytic enzymes (RNAase, DNAase, proteases, glycosidases, phosphatases) which on activation cause enzymatic digestion of cellular components and induce the nuclear changes (pyknosis, karyolysis and karyorrhexis) and hence cell death.

Serum estimation of liberated intracellular enzymes: Liberated enzymes leak across the abnormally permeable cell membrane into the serum, the estimation of which may be used as clinical parameters of cell death. For example, in myocardial infarction, estimation of elevated serum glutamic oxaloacetic transaminase (SGOT), lactic dehydrogenase (LDH), isoenzyme of creatine kinase (CK-MB), and more recently cardiac troponins (cTn) are useful guides for death of heart muscle.

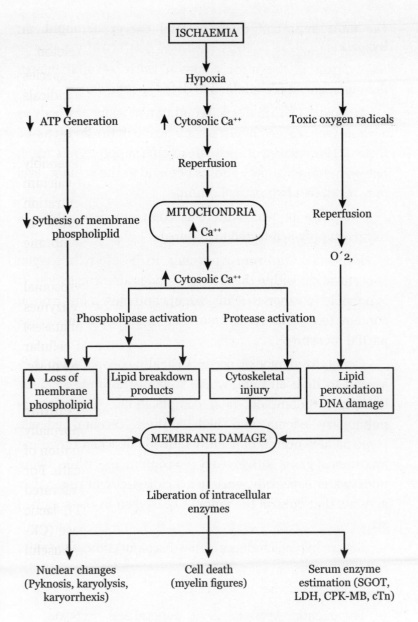

Fig. 10.5: Sequence of events in the pathogenesis of irreversible cell injury with hypoxia

The most important cause of vital energy derangement: Hypoxia

As hypoxia is the most common cause of vital energy derangement, it is explained in detail as follows.

Hypoxia is a pathological condition in which the body as a whole (generalized hypoxia) or a region of the body (tissue hypoxia) is deprived of adequate oxygen supply. A mismatch between oxygen supply and its demand at the cellular level may result in a hypoxic condition.

Hypoxia in which there is complete deprivation of oxygen supply is referred to as anoxia.

Hypoxia differs from hypoxemia. In the latter, the oxygen concentration within the arterial blood is abnormally low. It is possible to experience hypoxemia and have a low oxygen content (e.g., due to anemia) but maintain high oxygen partial pressure.

Generalized hypoxia occurs in healthy people when they ascend to high altitude, where it causes altitude sickness leading to potentially fatal complications: high altitude pulmonary edema and high altitude cerebral edema. Hypoxia also occurs in healthy individuals when breathing mixtures of gases with low oxygen content, e.g. while diving underwater especially when using closed-circuit rebreather systems that control the amount of oxygen in the supplied air.

Severe hypoxia induces a blue discolouration of the skin, called cyanosis.

Types of hypoxia

1. Hypoxemic hypoxia is a generalized hypoxia, an inadequate supply of oxygen to the body as a whole. The term 'hypoxemic hypoxia' specifies hypoxia caused

by low partial pressure of oxygen in arterial blood. Hypoxemic hypoxia may be due to:

- Low partial pressure of atmospheric oxygen such as found at high altitude or by replacement of oxygen in the breathing, made either accidentally as in the modified atmosphere of a sewer or intentionally as in the recreational use of nitrous oxide.

- A decrease in oxygen saturation of the blood caused by sleep apnoea or hypopnea.

- Inadequate pulmonary ventilation (e.g., in Chronic Obstructive Pulmonary Disease or Respiratory Arrest).

- Shunts in the pulmonary circulation or a right-to-left shunt in the heart. Shunts can be caused by collapsed alveoli that are still perfused or a block in ventilation to an area of the lung. Whatever the mechanism, blood meant for the pulmonary system is not ventilated and so no gas exchange occurs.

2   Anaemic hypoxia in which arterial oxygen pressure is normal, but total oxygen content of the blood is reduced.

- Hypoxia when the blood fails to deliver oxygen to target tissues.

- Carbon monoxide poisoning which inhibits the ability of haemoglobin to release the oxygen bound to it.

- Methaemoglobinaemia in which an abnormal version of haemoglobin accumulates in the blood.

3. Histotoxic hypoxia in which quantity of oxygen reaching the cells is normal, but the cells are unable to effectively

use the oxygen due to disabled oxidative phosphorylation enzymes. The effect of drinking alcoholic beverages is a common example.

4. Ischaemic or stagnant hypoxia in which there is a local restriction in the flow of otherwise well-oxygenated blood. The oxygen supplied to the region of the body is then insufficient for its needs. Examples are cerebral ischaemia, ischaemic heart disease, and intrauterine hypoxia, which is an important cause of perinatal death.

Local effects of hypoxia

Gangrene

Gangrene is a form of necrosis of tissue with superadded putrefaction. The type of necrosis is usually coagulative due to ischaemia.

1. Dry gangrene:

    This begins in the distal part of a limb due to ischaemia. Example is the dry gangrene in the toes and feet of an old patient due to arteriosclerosis.

    The gangrene spreads slowly upwards until it reaches a point where the blood supply is adequate to keep the tissue viable. A line of separation is formed at this point between the gangrenous part and the viable part.

    There is necrosis with smudging of the tissue. The line of separation consists of inflammatory granulation tissue.

2. Wet gangrene:

    This occurs in naturally moist tissues and organs such as the mouth, bowel, lung, cervix, vulva etc. Wet gangrene usually develops rapidly due to blockage of venous and less commonly arterial blood flow from thrombosis or embolism. There is coagulative necrosis with stuffing of affected part with blood. The affected part which is stuffed with blood, favors the rapid growth of putrefactive bacteria. The toxic products formed by bacteria are absorbed causing systemic manifestations of septicemia, and finally death. e.g., Diabetic foot, bed sores in a bed ridden patient.

3. Gas gangrene:

It is a special form of wet gangrene caused by gas-forming clostridia (gram – positive anaerobic bacteria) which gain entry into the tissues through open contaminated wounds, especially in the muscles, or as a complication of operation on colon which normally contains clostridia. Clostridia produce various toxins which produce necrosis and edema locally and are also absorbed producing profound systemic manifestations.

Necrosis

Necrosis (from the Greek word 'dead') is the name given to premature death of cells and living tissues caused by injury or disease. Hypoxia is the main cause of necrosis. Cells which die due to necrosis do not usually send the chemical signals to the immune system. This prevents nearby phagocytes from locating and engulfing the dead cells, leading to a buildup of dead tissue debris at the site of injury.

Cellular necrosis can be induced by a number of external sources, including injury, infection, cancer, infarction, poisons, and inflammation. For example, an infarction (blockage of blood flow to muscular tissue) causes necrosis of muscle tissue due to lack of oxygen to the affected cell, such as occurs in a myocardial infarction - a heart attack.

The sudden failure of one part of the cell triggers a so-called 'cascade of events'. In addition to the lack of chemical signals to the immune system, cells undergoing necrosis can release harmful chemicals into the surrounding tissue. In particular, cells contain small organelles called lysosomes, which are capable of digesting cellular material. Damage to the lysosome membrane can trigger release of the contained enzymes, destroying other parts of the cell. Worse, when these enzymes are released from the non-dead cell, they can trigger a chain reaction of further cell death. If a sufficient amount of adjacent tissue necrotizes, it is termed gangrene.

Necrosis typically begins with cell swelling, chromatin digestion, disruption of the plasma membrane and organelle. Late necrosis is characterized by extensive DNA hydrolysis, vacuolation of the endoplasmic reticulum, organelle breakdown, and cell lysis. The release of intracellular content after plasma membrane rupture is the cause of inflammation in necrosis.

Response to hypoxia

Vasoconstriction and vasodilatation

In most tissues of the body, the response to hypoxia is vasodilatation. By widening the blood vessels, the tissue allows greater perfusion.

By contrast, in the lungs, the response to hypoxia is vasoconstriction.

Effect of hypoxia on synaptic transmission

Neuronal excitability is also highly dependent on an adequate supply of oxygen. *Cessation of oxygen for only a few seconds can cause complete inexcitability of some neurons.* When the brain's blood flow is temporally interrupted, within 3 to 7 seconds, the person becomes unconscious.

The relation of vital force with hypoxia

As we term that vital force is nothing but oxygen energy and its supply to the body must be constantly maintained by the adequate respiration. Hypoxic condition can be explained through homeopathic miasms.

The degree of hypoxia is related to the miasms; psora, sycosis, tubercular, & syphilis. Anoxia i.e. the absence of oxygen in the cells is nothing but irreversible syphilitic condition.

Every type of pathology is related to the vital disturbance i.e. oxygen energy disturbance. It is the center of every pathological disorder.

Effects of foetal hypoxia

I have given importance to this subject specially to explain the role of vital energy since initiation of life.

The embryo's life begins where vital energy from the mother start flowing through the placenta.

The placenta forms a link between the foetus and mother. It is considered as an anchor for the growing foetus. It is not only the physical attachment between the foetus and mother, but also forms the physiological or vital connection between the two. The umbilical cord is the connecting link between the foetus and the placenta through which the foetal blood flows to and from the placenta. It consists of two arteries and two veins. The umbilical vein carries the oxygenated blood from the placenta to the foetus.

The placenta performs various functions like nutritive, excretory, respiratory, and endocrine. The major function of the placenta is to provide for diffusion of foodstuffs and oxygen from the mother's blood into the fetus's blood and diffusion of excretory products from the fetus back into the mother.

The exchange of respiratory gases between fetal blood and maternal blood occurs mostly because of pressure gradient. The partial pressure of oxygen in the maternal blood is 50 mm Hg. In the fetal blood the partial pressure of oxygen is 30 mm Hg. This pressure gradient of 20 mm Hg causes the diffusion of oxygen into the fetal blood. The haemoglobin in fetal blood has got 20 times more affinity for oxygen than the adult haemoglobin. The haemoglobin concentration is about 50% more in the fetal blood than in the mother's blood.

The importance of the vital force begins from the neonate's first breathe and if the neonate is unable to take the first breath, there will be a medical emergency. It will be hazardous to his life because the oxygen supply of the neonate is dependent on the mother's blood flow. When the umbilical cord is cut off after delivery, the neonate's respiratory system is spontaneously stimulated at the same second and the neonate starts crying and receives oxygen from the air to continue his independent life.

Birth Injuries

During delivery, there may be chances of obstruction of the neonate's airways (air passage) and the neonate may be unable to breathe spontaneously. As a result there may be irreversible damage of the neonatal brain cells i.e. neurons. And he will have to suffer lifelong disability. Here I would like to give you an example of cerebral palsy.

1. **Cerebral palsy** is caused by damage to one or more specific areas of the brain during periods of brain

development, commonly caused by hypoxia. The cerebrum is the largest part of the brain, responsible for higher mental faculties, sensations and voluntary muscle activities, and is usually affected by hypoxia. If the brain cells do not receive enough oxygen (vital energy) they may die. As brain cells are extremely sensitive to oxygen deprivation, some cells start dying in less than five minutes after their oxygen supply is cut off. As a result, brain hypoxia can kill or cause severe brain cell damage rapidly. When the neurons in this region die, proper signals can no longer be sent to the muscles under their control. This may result in poor muscle control and further exhibit the signs of cerebral palsy.

Most cerebral palsy cases that occur during birth happen because labor went on for too long. If the labor is allowed to continue, the fetus will suffer from lack of oxygen. If the heart rate changes rapidly, it's usually a sign of fetal distress, and the fetus needs to be delivered immediately. Sometimes the umbilical cord can twist or when the baby is too big, the cord can get squeezed too tightly. Oxygen deprivation here causes cerebral hypoxia, which results in cerebral palsy.

Another example is neonatal encephalopathy.

2. **Neonatal encephalopathy** is a clinically-defined synd-rome of disturbed neurological function that is noticed in the first few days of life of a term or near-term infant, and is manifested by difficulty with initiating and maintaining respirations, depression of tone and reflexes, subnormal level of consciousness, and often, seizures.

Neonatal encephalopathy that results from systemic hypoxemia and decreased cerebral perfusion leading to ischaemia is termed hypoxic-ischemic encephalopathy. Findings in near-term and term infants with hypoxic-ischemic encephalopathy include delay of spontaneous respirations at birth, seizures, altered level of consciousness, altered tone, decreased spontaneous movement, irregular respirations, apnea, poor or absent Moro's reflex, abnormal cry and suck, altered papillary responses, and stupor that develop in the first 72 hours after birth. Long-term morbidity and/or mortality after hypoxic-ischemic encephalopathy depend on the extent and severity of the injury.

Complications during delivery leading to hypoxia include large baby, twins, IUGR, asphyxia neonatorum etc.

Breech presentation, or prolonged labor sometimes require the use of forceps to safely deliver the baby, however, if proper medical procedures are not followed while using forceps, birth injuries such as nerve damage and cerebral hemorrhage leading to hypoxia and permanent infarction of the brain cells can result. Forceps used in child birth is permissible when baby appears to be in fetal distress, when the mother is having trouble pushing, or when the positioning of the baby in the birth canal is incorrect.

Correlation of vital energy (oxygen) with following factors of cell injury is explained in the chapter 14 'Vital energy derangement - Origin of pathology'.

Physical & Chemical injuries

Physical injuries

Many physical agents can damage cells and tissues. Examples of physical agents (including environmental agents) that can cause cellular or tissue injury include the following:

- Temperature extremes (hypothermic and hyperthermic injury).

- Changes in atmospheric pressure (blast injury, decompression sickness).

- Ionizing radiation (radiation injury).

- Nonionizing radiation (radio waves, microwaves).

- Illumination (light injury e.g., vision injury, skin cancer).

- Mechanical stresses (e.g., noise-induced hearing loss, overuse syndromes).

- Injuries caused by mechanical force may lead to a state of shock. Killing of cells by ionizing radiation is the result of direct formation of hydroxyl radicals from radiolysis of water. These hydroxyl radicals damage the cell membrane as well as may interact with DNA of the target cell

Chemical injuries

Many chemical agents can damage a cell. Examples include heavy metals (e.g., lead), carbon monoxide, ethanol, drugs, and complex toxins. Some of these chemicals injure cells directly (e.g., curare and cyanide). Others, when metabolized, produce a toxin that affects the cells (e.g., carbon tetrachloride).

The injury begins with a biochemical interaction. The interaction occurs between a toxic substance and an integral part of the cell's structure. Some drugs and toxins (e.g., Salicylate, certain venoms) affect the cellular membrane. This interaction can damage the plasma membrane. It can lead to increased permeability, cellular swelling, and irreversible cellular injury. Other toxins, such as carbon monoxide, mainly affect the cytochrome system found in the mitochondria. This leads to a halt in oxidative metabolism. Still other toxins affect the genetic material.

Microbial agents

Microorganisms, namely bacteria, viruses, fungi and parasites, are present everywhere - in the soil, water, and atmosphere and on the body surfaces, are responsible for a large number of infectious diseases in human beings.

Bacteria

Bacteria survive and damage the host in a variety of ways such as by generation of toxins (e.g. gas-forming anaerobes), by forming a slippery capsule that resists attachment to macrophages (e.g. pneumococci), by inhibition of fusion of phagocytic vacuoles with lysosomes (e.g. tubercle bacilli) etc.

Many bacteria that survive and multiply in the body produce toxins. These can injure or destroy cells and tissues.

The toxins take two forms: exotoxins and endotoxins.

Exotoxins are produced by a microorganism. Then they are excreted into the medium surrounding it. Exotoxins have highly specific effects. These effects are produced by the release of exotoxins as metabolic products during bacterial growth.

Endotoxins are complex molecules. They are contained in the cell walls of some bacteria.

When the body's defenses fail and microorganisms multiply in the blood, bacteremia develops. This may lead to septicemia, a severe systemic infection in which pathogens are present in the bloodstream. The endotoxins cause vasodilatation. This reduces blood pressure and oxygen delivery.

Viruses

Viral diseases are the most common cause of human illness. However, many of the viral infections remain asymptomatic while others produce viral disease. Another peculiar feature of viral infection is that a single etiologic agent may produce different diseases in the same host depending upon host immune response and age at infection. Viruses are essentially intracellular parasites. They can reproduce only by infecting the living cells of host tissue. Viruses usually consist of a protein coat (capsid) that encloses a core of nucleic acid. They often destroy the host cell. They have no organelles and therefore have no metabolism.

Viruses need nucleic acid either deoxyribonucleic acid [DNA] or ribonucleic acid [RNA] to replicate. Cells are thought to engulf the virus particles by surrounding them with part of the cell membrane. Once inside the cell, the virus loses the capsid and begins to replicate the viral nucleic acids. Some viruses cause the cell to burst. Others replicate without destroying the cell.

Fungi

Of the large number of known fungi, only a few are infective to human beings. Many of the human fungal infections are opportunistic i.e. they occur in conditions with impaired host immune mechanisms. Such conditions include defective neutrophil function, administration of corticosteroids, immunosuppressive therapy and immunodeficiency states (congenital and acquired).

Parasites

Diseases caused by parasites (protozoa and helminthes) are quite common and comprise a very large group of infestations in human beings. Parasites may cause disease due to their presence in the lumen of the intestine, due to infiltration into the blood stream, or due to their presence inside the cells.

Immunologic agents

Cellular membranes are damaged by direct contact with cellular and chemical components of the immune and inflammatory responses. These components include phagocytic cells (monocytes, neutrophils, and macrophages) and substances such as antibodies, lymphokines, complements, and proteases. If the cell membrane is injured or if the transport mechanism (which moves potassium into the cell and sodium out of it) begins to fail, intracellular water increases. This causes the cell to swell. If the swelling continues, the cell eventually may rupture.

Nutritional derangements

Cells need adequate amounts of essential nutrients to function normally. If the needed nutrients are not gained through the diet and taken to the cells, patho-physiological effects on the cells can occur. Damaging effects also can occur if the excessive amounts of nutrients are consumed and taken to the cells. When deficiency or excess is related to dietary intake, it can't be termed as disease entity but self induced as it depends on individual choice. Defective absorption and assimilation is related to disease entity and it definitely shows patho-physiological effects. Examples of conditions caused by injurious nutritional imbalances include obesity, scurvy, rickets, mal-absorption syndromes, etc.

Genetic factors

Genetic diseases results from a chromosomal abnormality or a defective gene. These genetic defects may be inherited. (An example of such a disease is sickle cell anemia). They also may result from spontaneous mutations. (An example is Down syndrome). Some genetic disorders can alter the cell's structure and function. Genetic disorders can cause changes in the structural or metabolic component of the specific target cells. Huntington disease and muscular dystrophy are examples of conditions caused by such disorders.

Psychological factors

Psychological factors can induce all kind of illness, not simply mental ones. They include conditions as essential hypertension, peptic ulcer, bronchial asthma etc. Medical illness as depression and schizophrenia also have biological component. Problems of drug addiction, alcoholism, and smoking which also have psychological background results in various organic diseases such as liver damage, chronic bronchitis, lung cancer, peptic ulcer, hypertension, ischemic heart disease, etc.

This psychological factor and its relation with oxygen are explained in detail in the chapter 13 'Oxygen (Vital Force) and its relation with emotions'.

CHAPTER 11

Mapping of Vital Energy Damages (Investigations and its use)

USE OF INVESTIGATIONS FROM HOMEOPATHIC POINT OF VIEW

PULSE-OXIMETRY

Mapping of Vital Energy Damages (Investigations and its use)

USE OF INVESTIGATIONS FROM HOMEOPATHIC POINT OF VIEW

Today's scientific research and development in medical and bio-engineering field gift us with abundant techniques and equipments of investigation methods. There are varied kind of investigations available which help us to reach the appropriate diagnosis; for instance X-ray, Electrocardiography, Echo-cardiogram, CT-Scan, MRI, PET-Scan, angiography, Colour Doppler, and various scopies (like Endoscopy, Colonoscopy), etc.

Different pathological investigations as haematology, tumor markers, and histopathology are at our easy disposal to help us know the diagnosis, and prognosis (i.e. progress and the gravity of vital damage).

The exact location and extent of damage of vital energy, as in Haemorrhage, Stroke, Embolism, Aneurysm,

Ischaemia, or Infarct can be easily visualized and noted with these investigations.

From Homeopathic point of view, these investigations are useful to understand the active miasm in a patient. In short all these investigations are aimed at mapping of extent of damage to vital energy (Oxygen energy).

Generalized measurement of oxygen saturation in human body (especially in emergency conditions) can be done with the help of Pulse oximetry.

PULSE-OXIMETRY

Pulse-oximeter helps to determine how well the patient is being oxygenated. They measure the transmission of red and near-infrared light through arterial beds. Haemoglobin absorbs red and infrared light waves differently when it is bound with oxygen (oxyhaemoglobin) and when it is not (reduced haemoglobin). Oxyhaemoglobin absorbs more infrared than red light. Reduced haemoglobin absorbs more red than infrared light. Pulse oximetry reveals arterial saturation by measuring this difference.

The percentage of haemoglobin saturated with oxygen is denoted as the Sao_2. It depends on a number of factors. These include the Pco_2, pH, temperature, and whether the haemoglobin is normal or altered. The lower range of normal for the Sao_2 is 93% to 95%. The upper range is 99% to 100%. Once the Sao_2 falls below 90% (corresponding to a Po_2 of 60 mm Hg), further decreases are associated with a marked decline in oxygen content.

Oxygen Saturation and Partial Pressure (Po_2):

With 90% saturation, Po_2 drops to 60 mm Hg.

With 75% saturation, Po_2 drops to 40 mm Hg.

With 50% saturation, Po_2 drops to 27 mm Hg.

All these equipments and techniques of investigation help us to reach the exact cause and character of the disease. It thus proves to be a boon which guides us for appropriate management of the patient.

Oxygen (Vital Force) and its Relation to Miasm

PSORA

SYCOSIS

TUBERCULAR

SYPHILIS

Oxygen (Vital Force) and its Relation to Miasm

According to homeopathic philosophy pathological state, remedy selection and the prognosis of the diseased person is mathematically dependent on the host miasm.

Miasm is the cause of disease that indicates the pathological state of a sick person.

There are four types of miasms, creating life threatening diseases in the human body i.e. psora, sycosis, tubercular and syphilis. They are well recognized miasms for the study in homeopathic science.

PSORA

Psoric miasm means physiological disturbance or dysfunctioning in the organism; e.g. Scabies which is an itching disorder of the superficial skin. Usually, in the healthy state the body does not express itching or irritation. If this irritation occurs in the different parts, it is expressed as symptoms and these symptoms indicate the disease. Most of the psoric diseases have tendency to recover rapidly without any medicine. They can be recovered with the help of immune response of the body. E.g., viral fever, viral gastritis, acute tonsillitis etc.

Psoric diseases present with functional disturbances with minor cell injury which is easily reversible, and it never presents with structural changes. Psoric miasm consists of simple, mild degree (I degree) lack of oxygen resulting in functional cellular disturbance.

The remaining miasms, sycosis, tubercular and syphilis are having actual structural changes due to reversible or irreversible cell injury. It is responsible for bad prognosis of the disease.

SYCOSIS

In the sycosis miasm the structural changes occur gradually, resulting in reversible or irreversible damage of the organ. E.g. Mitral stenosis - as a result of cell injury, structural changes take place in the mitral valve area causing thickening of the valve which gradually leads to stenosis. Simultaneously, due to the backpressures there is dilatation of the right atrium. Likewise, the sycotic miasm works in the body. The effect of sycosis is a manifestation of abnormal contraction, dilatation, indurations and tissue growth or hypertrophy.

Sycotic miasm is characterized by moderate degree of hypoxia or ischaemia (II degree) which is responsible for an abnormal cell behavior and cell injury. Hypoxia hampers the cellular metabolism which is responsible for the abnormal protein chain and the abnormal growth of the affected cells. If this state persists it causes neoplasm or tumor like growth.

So again moderate degree of hypoxia leads to irreversible cell damage, homeopathically we call it as sycosis miasm.

TUBERCULAR

This miasm is the connecting link between sycosis and syphilis. It represents with inflammation, degeneration, and atrophic changes at the cellular level and thus creates great disturbances in cellular functions with weakening the cell. For example, osteoarthritis, spondylosis, etc.

Tubercular miasm include the III degree oxygen derangement. Being the III degree hypoxic or ischemic state, the cell function is hampered to near complete and changes such as atrophy, degeneration, and emaciation are seen. In this miasmatic state, the cells try to survive with very less degree of oxygen. If this state persists, it gradually leads to complete destructive pathology that is syphilis.

SYPHILIS

Syphilitic miasm is characterized by infarction, necrosis and destruction of the suffering organ; for instance, myocardial infarction, cerebral stroke etc.

There is a great degree of vital derangement when syphilitic state progresses. This vital derangement is nothing but complete lack (or absence) of oxygen in the cell and in the suffering organ, creating metabolic threat of anaerobic energy. Thus the cell progresses towards death.

Syphilis indicates very low degree or the complete lack of oxygen (i.e. anoxia). This IV degree of oxygen derangement is a very serious situation as per the cell injury is concerned. The cell then gradually or suddenly progresses to destructive changes like infarction or necrosis that is premature cell death. Necrosis occurs as a destructive chain reaction; the tissue surrounding the necrotic cell also undergoes stepwise destructive changes and likewise group of cells (tissue) get affected. Further as it progresses, major part of the organ is involved creating functional disturbances thereby affecting the entire body.

Thus, all these miasmatic states occur in human being due to vital (oxygen) derangement.

Taking a short review of what is earlier mentioned in this book verifies that vital energy is nothing but oxygen energy. This will make us understand clearly that to what extent lack of oxygen in the healthy body is responsible for the varied types of dysfunctions leading to the cell injury.

The physician must understand the vital force well, to remove the vital disturbance of the body with the help of homeopathic remedy; as the properly selected Homeopathic remedy removes the obstacles that create derangement in cell metabolism and its oxygen supply.

Oxygen (Vital Force) and its Relation to Emotions

EMOTIONS

STRESS AND DISEASE

- Neuroendocrine regulation of stress
- Catecholamines
- Cortisol

EMOTIONAL DYSPNOEA

Oxygen (Vital Force) and its Relation to Emotions

Our guru Dr Samuel Hahnemann taught us that the state of mind (emotions) changes before the onset of disease. There is a great philosophy behind this thought. Here, he guides us that one must consider the patient with his physical & mental state (considering the patient as a whole) while prescribing the homeopathic medicine.

The meaning here to convey is that not only the mental state but abnormal sensations, symptoms and signs manifested during the illness must be considered as they in totality guide us to the actual state of the individual and to the correct remedy.

The human mind is a centre for emotions. Every emotional variation creates some change (good or bad) in the individual. Also, these variations express physically in the form of hormonal imbalance. If these changes persist for long; it leads to initiation of disease process.

As we relate lack of oxygen to physical signs and symptoms, likewise every abnormal thought leads to an abnormal breathing and ultimately result in lack of oxygen.

Let us now study in some more detail about the origin of emotions and its effects on physical level.

EMOTIONS

Cerebral cortex, limbic system and hypothalamus are responsible for the higher functions as memory, emotions etc.

Emotion is a mental state or a feeling such as fear, hate, love, anger, grief, or joy arising as a subjective experience rather than as a conscious thought which is controlled by the emotional cortex.

Limbic system (also called as basal region of brain) is particularly concerned with the affective nature of sensory sensations i.e. whether the sensations are pleasant or unpleasant. These emotional qualities are also called reward or punishment, or satisfaction or aversion. Electrical stimulation of certain limbic areas pleases or satisfies, whereas electrical stimulation of other regions causes terror, pain, fear, defense, escape reactions and all other elements of punishment.

Nerve signals in the brain stem activate the cerebral part of the brain in two ways:

1. By directly stimulating a background level of neuronal activity in wide areas of the brain.

2. By activating neurohormonal systems that release specific facilitory or inhibitory hormone - like neurotransmitter substances into selected areas of the brain.

We have learnt in the previous chapter that oxygen is responsible for the aerobic cellular metabolism and lack of oxygen causes hypoxia and further develops into cell injury.

During physical exercise or any emotional state more oxygen is required to meet increased metabolic requirement of the body. We have seen in previous chapter that, during exercise the muscular and cardiac activity increases, leading to rise in the ratio of demand and supply of oxygen. Likewise, during different emotional states lot of changes occur in the body from the biological point of view. The enzyme and hormone secretion increases resulting in increased cellular metabolic process and the oxygen consumption rate naturally increases. And to fulfill this oxygen requirement, the respiratory rate increases.

Respiration is primarily regulated for the metabolic and homeostatic purpose in the brainstem. However, breathing can also change in response to changes in emotions such as sadness, happiness, anxiety, or fear. Thus, the respiratory output is influenced by a complex interaction between the brainstem and higher centers of the brain, including the limbic system and cortical structures. In order to maintain physiological homeostasis normal rhythmic respiration (14-20 per minute) is a necessity.

STRESS AND DISEASE

As per the scientific view about stress, it is a specific response of the body to a demand, be it physical or psychological, perceived or real response of the cortical secretion or catecholamines (adrenaline + noradrenaline) or dopamine.

Prolonged emotional or psychological stress can result in physical illness. This type of illness can produce disturbances in three important areas; cognition, emotion, and behavior.

Neuroendocrine regulation of stress

During stress the alarm reaction is set off by the autonomic nervous system. This reaction is coordinated by the hypothalamus. The sympathetic nervous system is activated during the stress response. The hypothalamus triggers the pituitary gland to release adrenocorticotropic hormone into the bloodstream. This stress hormone stimulates the production of glucose. The hormone also increases the concentration of nutrients in the blood that provide energy. These nutrients are needed for the response to stress.

Adrenocorticotropic hormone also activates the adrenal glands for an intense sympathetic discharge of catecholamines i.e. adrenaline, noradrenaline and dopamine. These hormones cause the heart rate to increase, blood pressure to rise, and the pupils of the eyes to dilate, which improves vision. Together these hormones relax the bronchial tree for deeper breathing, increase blood sugar for total energy, slow the digestive process, and shift the blood supply to accommodate the clotting mechanism in case the body is wounded. After these physiological events, the body is ready for an emergency (fight or flight). The body can perform feats of strength and endurance far beyond its normal capacity. The alarm reaction takes only seconds.

Along with ACTH the pituitary gland also releases the hormones ADH, prolactin, growth hormone, and adrenocorticotropic hormone. ACTH in turn, stimulates the cortex of the adrenal gland to release cortisol.

Catecholamines

Catecholamines act by stimulating two major classes of receptors. These are alpha adrenergic receptors and beta adrenergic receptors. These two classes are further subcategorized into:

Alpha-1 receptors

Alpha-2 receptors

Beta-1 receptors

Beta-2 receptors

Alpha-1 receptors are postsynaptic. They are located on the effector organs (e.g., blood vessels, skeletal muscle). The main role of the alpha-1 receptors is to stimulate the contraction of smooth muscle.

The alpha-2 receptors are found on the presynaptic nerve endings. Stimulation of the alpha-2 receptors serves as a negative feedback mechanism by inhibiting further release of norepinephrine.

The beta-1 receptors are located mainly in the heart. Beta-2 receptors are located primarily in the bronchiolar and arterial smooth muscle. The beta receptors perform a number of functions. They stimulate the heart; dilate the bronchioles and the blood vessels in the skeletal muscle, brain, and heart; and aid in glycogenolysis.

Epinephrine activates both the alpha and beta receptors; norepinephrine mainly excites the alpha receptors.

Cortisol

Cortisol (hydrocortisone) circulates in the plasma. It mobilizes substances that are needed for cellular metabolism. The main metabolic effect of cortisol is the stimulation of gluconeogenesis. It also enhances the elevation of blood glucose. It does this by reducing glucose utilization. Cortisol also acts as an immunosuppressant; it reduces the reproduction of lymphocytes, particularly among the T lymphocytes. This, in turn, leads to a decrease in cellular immunity.

Cortisol also reduces the migration of macrophages into an inflamed area. It reduces phagocytes, partly by stabilizing the lysosomal membranes. This decrease in immune cell activity may be beneficial, because it prevents immune-mediated tissue damage. Two factors determine whether cortisol's effects are adaptive or destructive. These factors are the type of stress event and the length of exposure to the stressor.

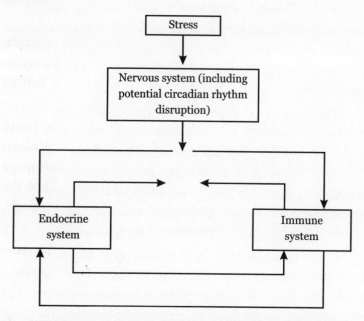

Fig. 13.1: Interaction of the emotional state, the central nervous system, endocrine system, and the body's defense against infection.

Stress has adverse effects on the mind and body. Some of them are as follows:

1. Increased heart rate, blood pressure, muscle tension, respiratory rate, oxygen consumption, blood sugar,

serum cholesterol, blood clotting, acid secretion in stomach, including secretion of cortisol and catecholamine.

2. Spasm of arteries.

3. Drying of saliva.

4. Bowel and bladder tone decreases.

Persistent emotional state causes bad effects on the body. Obviously, these circumstances lead to development of a disease state gradually.

Certain strong emotions create sudden impact on human body which may lead to sudden death. For example, sudden emotional turmoil may cause bronchospasm or coronary spasm leading to respiratory or cardiac arrest respectively.

Dyspnoea is a type of breathing difficulty. It also symbolizes mental anguish associated with inability to ventilate enough and satisfy the demand for oxygen. A common synonym is air hunger. In certain conditions the respiratory functions may be normal and still dyspnoea may be experienced because of an abnormal state of mind. This is called neurogenic or **emotional dyspnea**.

Many a times emotional effects and stress result in irregular, short, or labored breathing. This affects the oxygen intake by body. Health requires adequate oxygen supply and this can be attained by undertaking certain breathing exercises which maintain oxygen demand and supply ratio. And also the natural way of breathing should be smooth, easy and of abdominal type. It facilitates good oxygen intake → good metabolism → adequate oxygen energy production for day to day activities. It helps to control the effects of stress and avoid unnecessary hormonal secretions. Thus each appropriate breath of our life is very important for healthy and long life.

For the above mentioned reasons every physician should understand the importance of regular and rhythmic breathing and try to maintain the same in the patient.

Emotional stability that is balanced state of mind is a key to healthy life.

Vital Energy Derangement – Origin of Pathology

INTRODUCTION

ACUTE DISEASES

CHRONIC DISEASES

- Inflammation
  - —Stages of the inflammatory response
  - —Acute inflammation
  - —Chronic inflammation
- Haemodynamic disturbances
  - —Disturbances in the volume of the circulating blood
  - —Circulatory disturbances of obstructive nature
- Infectious and parasitic diseases
- Environmental and nutritional diseases
  - —Environmental Diseases
  - —Nutritional Diseases
  - —Effect of blood flow on gastrointestinal absorption
- Neoplasia
- Immunopathology
- Genetic diseases

Vital Energy Derangement – Origin of Pathology

Introduction

Most of the times, if the oxygen supply (vital energy) to a part or as a whole is altered, due to any kind of pathological or environmental reasons it will lead to mild, moderate or severe injury to the cell depending upon the duration of oxygen lack.

Each and every cell requires oxygenated blood for its activity i.e. aerobic respiration. Absence of oxygen will result in anaerobic metabolic activity which is a negligible source of energy and will never be enough for the energy requirement of the body.

When the microcirculation of tissue is damaged by any of the mechanical, chemical, micro-bacterial, environmental or by reactive oxygen species, aerobic metabolism is disturbed; short term anaerobic metabolism results which barely provide any energy and causes accumulation of harmful byproducts as lactic acid initiating the vital derangement. This results in mild to severe cell injury. Similar process occurs in varied general and systemic pathologies.

Lack of oxygen (vital energy) is thus responsible directly or indirectly for disturbance in cellular metabolism resulting in following enumerated pathologies which are the basic presentation of each and every disease:

1. Inflammation
2. Haemodynamic disorders
3. Infectious and parasitic diseases
4. Environmental and nutritional diseases
5. Neoplasia
6. Immunopathology
7. Genetic diseases

Depending upon the duration of cell injury disease process is divided into two conditions, acute diseases and chronic diseases.

Acute diseases

Acute conditions can be reversible or irreversible. For example Upper respiratory tract infection, routine Viral fever, Gastritis etc. are most of the times self limiting or easily treatable and are termed as reversible.

If complications such as necrosis, infarction results, it can be termed as irreversible. Here the cell injury process is rapid; the cell defense collapses immediately, leading to mitochondrial swelling, dysfunction, damage, and ischaemia leading to infarction; for example, Acute pneumonitis, Cerebral malaria, and Destructive dengue fever. Likewise, if this acute inflammatory disease condition occurs in gastrointestinal tract, for instance, food poisoning, or any kind of viral or bacterial infection occurring in intestine, there is a threat of severe vomiting and loose motions which creates severe dehydration, electrolyte imbalance, hypovolemia leading to hypotension, hypoxia and if untreated will lead to death.

In acute haemorrhagic conditions, the vital damage depends on

1. Amount of blood loss
2. Injury to vital organ
3. Alteration in the blood supply of the affected organ, example brain injury may cause sudden death due to hypoxia. Likewise spinal cord, cardiac, liver, renal, or any important organ injury, simply hampers the blood supply in this acute process, and if it is not restored or supplemented in time, hypoxia or infarction takes place leading to damage.

Chronic diseases

If this pathological process is delayed or slowed down, it will develop into a chronic disease condition; example, Osteoarthritis, Cervical spondylosis, Chronic renal failure, Liver cirrhosis, Parkinson's, Alzheimer, Hypertension, Diabetes mellitus, etc. In chronic condition there is long standing inflammation and mitochondrial swelling; this is the manifestation of sycosis miasm. If this cell injury process further persists, it will make mitochondria weaker i.e. a deranged state thereby reducing the oxygen carrying capacity of mitochondria. This is manifestation of tubercular miasm. If this process continues cell will land in total dysfunction with changes as calcification of mitochondria and the resulting total oxygen lack will cause, cell death; indicating expression of syphilitic miasm. Chronic diseases are thus characterized by cellular damages such as degeneration, calcification, fibrosis etc. In chronic diseases the prognosis depends on severity of damage and amount of viable tissue available.

Inflammation

It is a local response of living tissues to injury due to any agent. It is a body defense reaction in order to eliminate or limit the spread of injurious agent as well as to remove the consequent necrosed cells and tissues.

Rubor (redness), calor (heat), dolor (pain), tumor (swelling) and loss of function are the five cardinal signs of inflammation.

Stages of the inflammatory response

The inflammatory response may be divided into three separate stages; these are:

1. The cellular response to injury
2. The vascular response to injury
3. Phagocytosis

Cellular response to injury

Metabolic changes occur with any type of cellular injury. The most common primary effect of cellular injury is damage to the cell's aerobic metabolism and ATP-generating process (oxidative phosphorylation). This leads to a decrease in energy reserves. When the energy sources are depleted, the sodium - potassium pumps can no longer work effectively. The cell begins to swell as sodium ions accumulate. The organelles in the cell also swell. This swelling, along with increasing acidosis, leads to further impairment of enzyme function. It also leads to further deterioration of the cell's membranes. In time, the membranes of the cellular organelles begin to leak. The release of hydrolytic enzymes by the lysosomes contributes further to cellular destruction and autolysis. As the cellular contents are dissolved by enzymes, the inflammatory response is stimulated in surrounding tissues.

Vascular response to injury

After cellular injury, localized hyperemia (an increase in organ blood flow) develops as the surrounding arterioles, venules, and capillaries dilate. The associated increase in filtration pressure and capillary permeability causes fluid to leak from the vessels. It leaks into the interstitial space. This creates edema. Leukocytes (particularly neutrophils and monocytes) begin to collect along the vascular endothelium. As a result of the release of chemo-tactic factors (chemicals that attract white cells to the site of inflammation); they soon migrate to the injured tissue.

Phagocytosis

Phagocytosis is the process by which leukocytes engulf, digest, and destroy pathogens. The circulating macrophages are also responsible for clearing the injured area of dead cells and other debris. Intracellular phagocytosis is the ingestion of bacteria and dead cell fragments. It occurs at the site of tissue invasion. It may extend into the general circulation if the infection becomes systemic. Intracellular phagocytosis stimulates the release of chemicals that induce lysis of the leukocytes. These leukocytes combine with dead organisms, proteins, and fluid to form inflammatory exudates (commonly known as pus). This exudate is a by-product of the inflammatory process associated with bacterial infection.

Acute inflammation

Acute inflammation may be characterized by both local and systemic effects. Local responses include vascular changes (vasodilatation and increased vascular permeability) and the formation of exudates. Systemic responses include fever, leukocytosis, and an increase in circulating plasma proteins.

Chronic inflammation

Chronic inflammation lasts two weeks or longer. It can result from a persistent acute inflammatory response. This type of response may be caused by bacterial contamination by a foreign body (e.g. wood splinter, glass), persistent infection, or continued exposure to an antigen. If the inflammatory process is severe or prolonged, the body attempts to repair or replace tissue that has been damaged. To perform this repair, the body produces connective tissue fibres and new blood vessels. If the area of tissue destruction is large, scar tissue forms.

The main features of chronic inflammation are:

1. Infiltration by mononuclear cells – phagocytes and lymphoid cells specially macrophages.

2. Tissue destruction or necrosis by activated macrophages.

3. Proliferative changes.

Haemodynamic disturbances

Haemodynamic disturbance is a major cause for the vital (central) disturbances i.e. oxygen energy disturbance.

The meaning of central disturbance is oxygen imbalance causing cellular, tissue and thereby organ damage.

Haemodynamic disturbances are considered under two broad headings:

1. Disturbances in the volume of the circulating blood:

These include hyperemia and congestion, hemorrhage and shock.

2. Circulatory disturbances of obstructive nature:

These are thrombosis, embolism, ischaemia, and infarction.

Disturbances in the volume of the circulating blood

Hyperaemia and congestion

In hyperaemia and congestion there is increased volume of blood within dilated vessels of an organ or tissue, fulfilling the increase demand of oxygen.

The dilatation of veins and capillaries due to impaired venous drainage results in venous congestion (stasis of deoxygenated blood). e.g. chronic venous congestion of lung occurs in left heart failure, especially in left ventricular failure. Here, the alveolar septa are widened due to presence of interstitial edema as well as due to dilated and congested capillaries. Rupture of dilated and congested capillaries may result in minute intra-alveolar hemorrhages. The breakdown of erythrocytes liberates hemosiderin pigment which is taken up by alveolar macrophages, present in the alveolar lumina.

In this condition, the central disturbance occurs due to cellular swelling. It leads to intracellular disturbance and the raised intracellular pressure which creates mitochondrial dysfunction.

Once the mitochondrion is injured, there will be permanent, irreversible cell injury. This condition occurs due to inactivity of cardiac muscles leading to low cardiac output.

Inactivity of cardiac muscles is a condition where

cardiac muscles are not getting proper oxygen supply e.g. Cardiomyopathy, endocarditis.

The gradual development of this disease pathology is very similar to manifestation of miasms i.e. psora, sycosis, tubercular or syphilis.

Haemorrhage

Haemorrhage is the escape of blood from a blood vessel. Extravasation of blood into the tissues with resultant swelling is known as hematoma. Large extravasations of blood into the skin and mucous membranes are called ecchymosis. Purpuras are small areas of haemorrhages into the skin and mucous membrane, whereas petechiae are minute pinhead sized haemorrhages.

Causes of haemorrhages are:

- Trauma to vessel wall
- Spontaneous haemorrhage
- Inflammatory lesions of the vessel wall
- Neoplastic invasion
- Vascular diseases
- Elevated pressure within the vessels

Any haemorrhagic condition is abundant blood loss which means loss of vital energy. If the haemorrhagic condition does not stop within a few minutes, the respective cell and tissue undergo damage due to necrosis and infarction.

The damage of the disease depends on the amount of blood loss, the speed of blood loss and the site of the haemorrhage.

Shock

Shock is a clinical state of cardiovascular collapse characterized by an acute reduction of effective circulating blood volume and an inadequate perfusion of cells and tissues. Shock results in rapid vital derangement and may cause sudden death. The end result is hypotension, cellular hypoxia and, if uncompensated, may lead to impaired cellular metabolism and death.

Reduction in effective circulating blood volume may be from actual loss of blood or by decreased cardiac output causing decreased supply of oxygen to organs and tissues hence tissue anoxia and shock ensues. The morphologic changes in shock are due to hypoxia resulting in degeneration and necrosis in various organs. The major organs affected are the brain, heart, lungs, and kidneys.

Classification of shock:

1. Hypovolemic shock: For e.g. haemorrhage, burns, severe or prolong diarrhoea
2. Cardiogenic shock
3. Neurogenic shock
4. Anaphylactic shock
5. Septic shock

Circulatory disturbances of obstructive nature

Thrombosis

In some pathological conditions supply of vital energy to the part is blocked. Likewise, in thrombosis the process of formation of solid mass in circulation from the constituents of flowing blood lead to ischaemic injury, which may subsequently result in infarction and thromboembolism.

1. Arterial thrombi are formed following endothelial cell injury as in atherosclerosis and produce ischaemia and infarction. Arterial thrombi cause ischaemic necrosis of the deprived part (infarct) which may lead to gangrene.

For e.g. Sudden death may occur following thrombosis of coronary artery.

2. Venous thrombi are formed following venous stasis and it may cause various effects as thromboembolism, oedema of area drained; poor wound healing, skin ulcers, painful thrombosis of the veins, etc.

Embolism

Embolism is the process of partial or complete obstruction of some part of the cardiovascular system by any mass carried in the circulation; the transported intravascular mass detached from its site of origin is called an embolus. Most usual forms of emboli (90%) are thromboemboli, which means originating from thrombi or their parts detached from the vessel wall.

These may arise in the arterial or venous circulation.

1. Arterial emboli: The effects of arterial emboli are Infarction, Gangrene, Arteritis and Mycotic aneurysm, Myocardial Infarction and sudden death.

2. Venous emboli: The most significant effect of venous embolism is Obstruction of Pulmonary Arterial Circulation leading to Pulmonary embolism.

In pulmonary embolism, obstruction of relatively small sized pulmonary arterial branches may result in pulmonary infarction and massive embolus may cause instantaneous death.

Ischaemia

Along with hypoxia, ischaemia is also an important cause of cell injury.

Ischaemia is defined as deficient blood supply to part of a tissue.

Ischaemia (Greek *isch-* is restriction, *haema* is blood) is a restriction in blood supply, generally due to factors in the blood vessels, with resultant damage or dysfunction of tissue.

Mechanism

Ischaemia is an absolute or relative shortage of the blood supply to an organ, i.e. a shortage of oxygen, glucose and other blood-borne fuels. A relative shortage means the mismatch of blood supply (oxygen delivery) and blood demand for an adequate metabolism of tissue. Ischaemia results in tissue damage because of lack of oxygen and nutrients. Ultimately, this can cause severe damage because of the potential for a build-up of metabolic wastes.

Ischaemia can also be described as an inadequate flow of blood to a part of the body, caused by constriction or blockage of the blood vessels supplying it. Ischaemia of heart muscle produces angina pectoris.

This can be due to:

1. Hypoglycemia (sudden fall in fuel supply)
2. Tachycardia (abnormally rapid beating of the heart)
3. Atherosclerosis (lipid-laden plaques obstructing the lumen of arteries)
4. Hypotension (low blood pressure, e.g. in septic shock, heart failure)
5. Thromboembolism (blood clots)
6. Outside compression of a blood vessel, e.g. by a tumor or in the case of superior mesenteric artery syndrome
7. Embolism (foreign bodies in the circulation, e.g. amniotic fluid embolism)

8. Sickle cell disease (abnormally shaped red blood cells)

9. Localized extreme cold, such as by frostbite, ice, or improper cold compression therapy

Consequences

Since oxygen is mainly bound to haemoglobin in red blood cells, insufficient blood supply causes tissue to become hypoxic, or, if no oxygen is supplied at all, anoxic. In very aerobic tissues such as heart and brain, at body temperature necrosis due to ischaemia usually takes about 3 to 4 hours before becoming irreversible. However, complete cessation of oxygenation of such organs for more than 20 minutes typically results in irreversible damage.

The heart, the kidneys, and the brain are among the organs that are the most sensitive to inadequate blood supply. Ischaemia in brain tissue, for example due to stroke or head injury, causes a process called the ischemic cascade to be unleashed, in which proteolytic enzymes, reactive oxygen species, and other harmful chemicals damage and may ultimately kill brain tissue.

Infarction

Infarction is death of tissue that results from deprivation of its blood supply. This definition is very close to the miasmatic concept of syphilis.

An area of tissue in an organ or part undergoes necrosis following cessation of the blood supply. This may result from blockage of the tissue's blood supply. The supplying artery may be blocked by an obstruction (e.g. an embolus, thrombus, or atherosclerotic plaque), may be mechanically compressed (e.g. Tumor, Volvulus, or Hernia), ruptured by trauma (e.g. Atherosclerosis), or vasoconstrictor (e.g. Cocaine vasoconstriction leading to Myocardial Infarction).

Infarction is a complication of thrombosis. In thrombosis, there is occlusion of lumen of the blood vessel. The solid mass of platelets, red cells, or clots obstructs the blood vessel causing derangement of the vital force (i.e. hampered supply of oxygen). Sometimes this thrombus totally occludes the vessel causing infarct and instant cell death. For example, myocardial infarction occurs with a sudden and total blockage or near blockage of blood flowing through an affected coronary artery to an area of heart muscle. This blockage results in ischaemia, injury, and necrosis to the area of the myocardium distal to the occlusion. Other factors that may lead to myocardial infarction include coronary spasm, coronary embolism, severe hypoxia, hemorrhage into a diseased arterial wall, and reduced blood flow after any type of shock.

Atherosclerosis

It is a progressive occlusive lesion causing reduced flow of vital energy.

Atherosclerotic vascular disease may manifest as Coronary Heart Disease (Angina, Myocardial Infarction), cerebrovascular disease (Stroke and Transient Ischaemic attack), or peripheral vascular disease (Buerger's disease etc.)

Atherosclerosis is a progressive inflammatory disorder of the arterial wall that is characterized by focal lipid-rich deposits of atheroma that remain clinically silent until they become large enough to impair arterial perfusion or until ulceration or disruption of the lesion result in thrombotic occlusion or embolization of the affected vessel. These mechanisms are common to entire vascular tree. Oxygen radicals are said to play important role for plaque formation.

In advanced atherosclerosis any mechanical stress may lead to erosion, fissuring, or rupture of the plaque surface leading to platelet aggregation and thrombosis occluding the arterial lumen. This type of plaque event may cause partial or complete obstruction at the site of the lesion and or distal embolization resulting in infarction or ischaemia of the organ.

Angina is the symptom complex caused by transient myocardial ischaemia. It occurs whenever there is an imbalance between myocardial oxygen supply and demand.

Infectious and Parasitic Diseases

When oxygen level (vital energy) in the body becomes extremely low for too long period of time, the body becomes a perfect feeding ground for every sort of harmful bacteria, viruses, fungus, parasites, and other infectious agents. In short, most infectious agents simply cannot live in an oxygen rich environment. Most infections micro-organisms merely cannot colonize and proliferate there. The high oxygen content of our body oxidizes them along with disease causing byproduct.

Microorganisms after entering the body may spread further through the phagocytes, blood vessels, and lymphatics. Endotoxins are released on lysis of the bacterial cells while exotoxins are secreted by bacteria.

Environmental and Nutritional Diseases

Environmental Diseases

For survival of mankind, it is important to prevent depletion of ozone layer in the outer space from pollutants such as chlorofluorocarbons, nitrogen dioxide (NO_2) produced in abundance by day-to-day activities on our planet earth due to industrial effluent and automobile exhausts.

Air pollution

There are some pollutants prevalent in certain industries, such as coal, dust, silica, asbestos etc. Others are general pollutants present widespread in the atmosphere such as sulphur dioxide, carbon monoxide.

Tobacco Smoking

Tobacco smoking is the most prevalent and preventable cause of disease and death.

Here, several factors decrease respiratory efficiency as follows:

1. Nicotine constricts terminal bronchioles and this decreases airflow into and out of the lungs.

2. Carbon monoxide in smoke binds to haemoglobin and reduces its oxygen carrying capability.

3. Irritants in smoke cause increased fluid secretion by the mucosa of the bronchial tree and swelling of the mucosal lining which both impede airflow into and out of the lungs.

4. Irritants in smoke also inhibit the movement of cilia in the lining of the respiratory system. Thus, excess fluids and foreign debris are not easily removed.

5. Smoking also leads to destruction of elastic fibers in the lungs and emphysema. These changes cause collapse of small bronchioles and trapping of air in alveoli at the end of exhalation; causing less efficient gas exchange.

Many environmental (the air, sun, dust, etc) and industrial agents such as tobacco, smoke, stored food products, dietary trace element, additives, some metals, pesticides, ozone, NO_2 will produce an oxidative stress response with antioxidant defense system causing oxidative damage to tissues.

Carbon monoxide

It is one of the prevalent pollutant (from automobile exhaust, tobacco, etc.) causing systemic oxygen deprivation of tissues. This is because haemoglobin has about 200 times higher affinity for carbon monoxide than for oxygen.

Likewise, cyanide in the environment is released by combustion of plastic, silk, etc.

It is very toxic chemical and kills the cell by blocking cellular respiration by binding to mitochondrial cytochrome oxidase.

Physical agents

Physical agents like ionizing radiation has three types of effects on cells:

1. Somatic effects which cause acute cell killing
2. Genetic damage by mutations causing genetic defects
3. Malignant transformation of cells

Radiation - induced cell death is mediated by radiolysis of water in the cell with generation of toxic hydroxyl radicals.

As we see in general, due to poisonous gases, air pollution creates bad effects not only on the respiratory organ but also on cellular respiration. This causes dysfunction of mitochondrial activity and the pathological changes occur from this moment which end-up into reversible or irreversible cell injury and death.

Chemical factors

Oxygenation proponents follow the lines of Koch and Warburg. They claim that toxins which adulterate processed food, the environment, and medications damage the oxidative metabolism of normal cells which then regress into defective metabolism.

Nutritional Diseases

For healthy functioning of the cell, cell organelles, especially mitochondria which are the vital energy storage unit require adequate amount of nutrients. Proteins, fats, carbohydrates, vitamins, minerals, and water are the six basic groups of essential nutrients responsible for every cellular foundation and their harmonious functions.

Lack or excess of any type of essential nutrients creates nutritional diseases and the cell becomes ill; obviously the body will not receive the sufficient amount of vital energy.

There are two types of nutritional deficiencies:

1. Primary: This is due to either the lack or decreased amount of essential nutrients in diet. As mentioned previously when deficiency or excess is related to dietary intake, it can't be termed as disease entity but self induced as it depends on individual choice.

2. Secondary or conditioned deficiency: It is a malnutrition occurring as a result of the various factors.

   • Interference with ingestion e.g., Neuropsychiatric illness, anorexia, alcoholism, food allergy.

   • Interference with absorption e.g. in Hyper-motility of the gut, achlorhydria, biliary disease.

   • Interference with utilization e.g. in Liver dysfunction, hypothyroidism, malignancy.

   • Increased excretion e.g. in Lactation, perspiration, polyuria.

- Increased nutritional demand e.g. in Fever, pregnancy, hyperthyroidism.

With the help of following information, I want to explain that lack of oxygen is responsible for nutritional disorders related to absorption.

Effect of blood flow on gastrointestinal absorption

Under normal conditions, the blood flow in each area of the gastrointestinal tract, as well as in each layer of the gut wall, is directly related to the level of local activity. For instance, during active absorption of nutrients, blood flow in the villi and adjacent regions of the sub-mucosa is increased as much as eightfold. Likewise, blood flow in the muscle layers of the intestinal wall increases with increased motor activity in the gut. For instance, after a meal, the motor activity, secretory activity, and absorptive activity all increase; likewise, the blood flow increases greatly but then decreases back to the resting level over another 2 to 4 hours.

'Countercurrent' blood flow in the villi: The arterial flow into the villus and the venous flow out of the villus are in directions opposite to each other, and that the vessels lie in close opposition to each other. Because of this vascular arrangement, much of the blood oxygen diffuses out of the arterioles directly into the adjacent venules without ever being carried in the blood to the tips of the villi. As much as 80 per cent of the oxygen may take this short circuit route and therefore not be available for local metabolic functions of the villi. The reader will recognize that this type of countercurrent mechanism in the villi is analogous to the countercurrent mechanism in the vasa recta of the kidney medulla.

Under normal conditions, this shunting of oxygen from the arterioles to the venules is not harmful to the villi, but in disease conditions in which blood flow to the gut becomes greatly curtailed, such as in circulatory shock, the oxygen deficit in the tips of the villi can become so great that the villus tip or even the whole villus suffers ischaemic death and can disintegrate. Therefore, for this reason and others, in many gastrointestinal diseases the villi become seriously blunted, leading to greatly diminished intestinal absorptive capacity.

Every nutritional disorder leads to decreased energy production and maintenance. Because of this, the mitochondrial function gets hampered and cell is unable to consume proper oxygen. Obviously, this condition weakens the body immunity and may create ground for multiple infections.

Neoplasia

As per the homeopathic philosophy, neoplasia is a representation of sycosis miasm. Whenever, there is a lack of oxygen in the human body, cells starts abnormal behavior. If this state persists, gradually, the cell undergoes uncontrolled growth and tumour forms; be it benign or malignant. This fact supports Dr Samual Hahnemann's thought that 'derangement of vital force (oxygen), causes central disturbance which leads to diseased state.'

Neoplasia means new growth; the new growth produced is called tumor or neoplasm, but the satisfactory definition is 'a mass of tissue formed as a result of abnormal, excessive, uncoordinated, autonomous, and purposeless proliferation of cells.' Neoplasm may be 'benign' when they are slow growing and localized. They become 'malignant' when they proliferate independently and rapidly.

How this abnormal growth which occur in human body, causes threatening effects, is really shocking.

World famous noble prize winner Dr Laureate Otto Warburg said that the normal cells would become irreversibly cancerous, if the environment they rested in had their oxygen levels lowered by 35% for 48 hrs. Basically, the oxygen is required for aerobic metabolism in each and every cell. Lack of oxygen or hypoxia causes immediate metabolic disorders for example, in ATP energy production – glucose and oxygen is responsible. At the same time, not only for the energy production, but also metabolism of proteins and fats require oxidative phosphorylation. Obviously, the lack of oxygen for few minutes can be responsible for cellular metabolic dysfunction. If this state persists, it leads to irreversible metabolic cell dysfunction and abnormal protein production. It then causes dysfunction in DNA and RNA reactions (synthesis). Gradually it leads to abnormal cell metabolism and abnormal growth of the suffering cell. *Thus oxygen imbalance results in cancerous conditions.* Further tumor hypoxia is associated with poor prognosis for patients with various cancers often resulting in increase in metastasis. For example, exposure to hypoxia increases the ability of breast cancer to invade through extra cellular matrix.

Aerobic metabolism- ATP (energy) from
glucose, fats, proteins require oxidative phosphorylation

↓

If lack of oxygen

↓

Cellular metabolic dysfunction

↓ If O_2 lack persist

Cell damage

Due to accumulation of waste products

↓ O_2 lack still persist

Irreversible damage to cell

↓

Abnormal protein production

↓

Dysfunction in DNA & RNA synthesis

↓

Abnormal cell metabolism

↓

Abnormal growth of the suffering cells
i.e. Cancerous growth

Fig. 14.1: How Oxygen imbalance can result in cancerous conditions

Immunopathology

Vital energy (oxygen) plays an important role in the immune pathological conditions. Like other diseases, immune deficiency diseases also occurs due to insufficient oxygen supply to the immune cell's which create some defective components of immune systems; it results in immune cell's failure to function properly and is unable to produce required antibodies.

Immunity is the resistance of body against the pathogenic agents. It is the ability of the body to resist all types of bacteria, viruses, and toxic substances etc. which enter the body.

It is of two types:

1. **Innate immunity:** This is the inborn capacity of the body to resist any invader in general. It works as follows:

   • Activities of white blood cells and tissue macrophages which destroy the foreign bodies by phagocytes.

   • The enzymes of G.I.T. and the acid in stomach which destroy the toxic substances or organism entering digestive tract through food.

   • Protective function of skin against bacteria or other organisms and against ultra-violet rays.

   • Lysozome and some polypeptides which destroy or inactivate the bacteria.

2. **Acquired immunity:** It is the resistance developed in the body against any specific foreign body like bacteria, viruses, toxins or tissues transplanted from other's body. The acquired immunity is developed by the lymphocytes.

There are two types of acquired immunity - Cellular and Humoral immunity.

Cellular immunity is by the activation of T-lymphocytes, which destroy the organisms entering the body. All the lymphocytes are released in the circulation.

The cellular immunity is carried by the T lymphocytes. It develops when an antigen or antigenic material from the invading microbial or nonmicrobial cell is exposed to the T lymphocytes. This is done by antigen presenting cells.

There are two types of antigen presenting cells in the body:

Macrophages and dendritic cells.

The macrophages are the large phagocytic cells, which digest the invading organisms to release the antigen.

Humoral immunity is by the activation of B lymphocytes which fight against the invading organism by producing antibodies. This type of immunity plays an important role in the defense mechanism against the bacteria.

Oxygen depletion weakens our immune system which leads to varied infections, cell damage, growths, inflamed joints, etc. with toxic material build-up in blood and leads to premature aging. Low oxygen allows damaged cells to multiply and form growths in our bodies.

The B lymphocytes are proliferated into 2 types namely plasma cells and memory cells. The plasma cells produce antibodies. The rate of antibodies production is very high in plasma cell. Each plasma cell produces 2,000 micron per second. The antibodies are produced into the lymph and then transported into the circulation. The antibodies are produced till the end of life span of each plasma cell. If the plasma cell does not receive the appropriate amount of oxygen molecules for their maintenance and function, the production of the antibodies rate will be naturally decreased. Obviously, if the body defense system is collapsed, it would be the opportunity for bacteria and viruses to enter in the system, and do the further destruction.

For instance, AIDS (Acquired Immune Deficiency Syndrome).

AIDS results from infection by HIV virus (Human immunodeficiency virus).The initial response to HIV invasion is a modest decline in the number of circulating T4 cells. Infected people experience a brief flu-like illness, with chills and fever, but the immune system fights back by making antibodies against HIV and the number of circulating T4 cells recovers nearly to normal. Although infected people test positive for HIV antibodies, they typically have few clinical signs or symptoms and do not yet have AIDS.

Over the next 2-10 years, further lack of oxygen results from weakened immunity and psychological impact (depression, guilt, embarrassment, isolation etc.) due to social stigma. The virus slowly destroys the T4 cell population in lymphatic tissues throughout the body. As immune responses are weakened, the patient develops certain diseases. At this point, the diagnosis of AIDS is made.

AIDS infection occur when the glycoprotein from HIV binds to the surface receptors of T-lymphocytes, monocytes, macrophages and dendrite cells leading to destruction of these cells. This leads to slow and progressive decrease in immune function.

Virus contains an enzyme called reverse transcriptase. HIV utilize this enzyme and convert its own viral RNA into viral DNA with the help of host cell DNA itself. Now the viral DNA gets incorporated and prevents the normal activity of the host cell DNA. At the same time, the HIV increase in number inside the host body. The infected host cell ruptures and release more number of HIV viruses into the blood stream.

Thus if cell gets proper oxygen supply, the affected patient will be maintained in carrier stage of HIV and will not progress towards the AIDS stage.

Genetic Diseases

Genetic disorder is unpredictable as per the modern science is concerned. There are multiple reasons and factors involved in it. After lots of experiments and research, the various aspects of the subject are unknown as to what are the exact causes of genetic changes and mutations.

But today, we go through it by homeopathic philosophical point of view that, *'the basic and centralized theme behind every pathology is the disturbance or lack of vital energy'*.

The great majority of the genetic disorders are caused by the defect in the nuclear genome. However, most of the significant diseases are the result of mitochondrial mutations. Free radically mediated cell injury is also responsible for genetic disorders.

It is proved that each and every cell requires an adequate amount of oxygen at every second. If the cell could not receive enough amounts of oxygen it immediately results in disturbed functions. If hypoxia persists the cell starts malfunctioning. There is accumulation of waste products due to altered metabolism causing defective protein production. This eventually affects the DNA and RNA synthesis. The protein sequence of the genes is disturbed leading to change in genetic code. These cells thus continue to survive with their disturbed functions.

Due to malfunctioning, the cell does not get proper signaling and intracellular messages. It starts living individually and produces or generates new cell by cell division.

As mentioned earlier genetic diseases result from mitochondrial mutation. The patho-physiology of mitochondrial DNA (mtDNA) diseases is caused by increased cell death and dysfunction due to the accumulation of mutations to mtDNA. While the disturbance of oxidative phosphorylation is central to mtDNA diseases, many other factors, such as Ca(2+) dyshomeostasis increased oxidative stress and defective turnover of mitochondrial proteins, may also contribute.

According to Dr Samuel Hahnemann's theory of miasm and concept of vital force it is proved that the mitochondrial disturbance initially creates psoric state, in the living organisms. But the degree of mitochondrial dysfunction is also comparatively related to expressions of sycosis, tubercular, and syphilis miasms.

The complete dysfunction of the mitochondria leads to irreversible cell injury or cell destruction creating a picture similar to that of syphilitic miasm, and only homeopathic medicines have the potential to act on the intracellular structures to reestablish the dysfunction of the mitochondria.

CHAPTER 15

Oxygen and its Relation with Homeopathic Medicine

NERVOUS SYSTEM DIVISIONS

- Receptors

METHOD OF PREPARATION OF DYNAMIC MEDICINE

DRUG PROVING / ACTION OF HOMEOPATHIC MEDICINE ON HEALTHY HUMAN BEING

ACTION OF HOMEOPATHIC MEDICINE ON DISEASED PERSON

Oxygen and its Relation with Homeopathic Medicine

The human body is an extremely amazing functional frame work. The information whether it is related with food, weather, enemies like bacteria, viruses, toxins, thermal changes, destructive rays (ultra violet rays), different kinds of sounds and also different kinds of colours are received by body through thousands of trillion receptors. Likewise, the multiple signals about the present atmosphere and surroundings are received by our body. These signals received by receptors are transmitted to brain via nerves.

Every cell has its own receptors. The functioning of various cellular systems is based on receptors. Although these receptors are responsible for the intra and extra cellular chemical activities, each and every cell of our body is connected to the brain with individual cellular activities. There are different types of receptors which are having their own function and which play an important role as a bridge between the intracellular activities and central nervous system.

For example, to carry out any job through the brain, the neurons create stimulation through dendrites to cell receptors and appropriate action would be taken accordingly.

Before understanding the action of homeopathic medicine on human body, the understanding of nervous system physiology is immensely important.

Nervous system divisions

The two principle divisions of the nervous system are the Central Nervous System (CNS) and the Peripheral Nervous System (PNS).

The CNS consists of the brain and spinal cord. Within the CNS many different kinds of incoming sensory information is integrated and correlated, thoughts and emotions are generated, and memories are formed and stored. Most nerve impulses that stimulate the muscles to contract and glands to secrete originate in the CNS.

The CNS is connected to sensory receptors, muscles, and glands in peripheral parts of the body by the PNS. The PNS consists of cranial nerves that arise from the brain and spinal nerves that emerge from the spinal cord. Some parts of these nerves carry impulses into the CNS while other portions carry impulses out of the CNS.

The input component of the PNS consists of nerve cells called sensory or afferent neurons. They conduct nerve impulses from sensory receptors in various parts of the body to the CNS and end within the CNS. The output component consists of nerve cells called motor or efferent neurons. They originate within the CNS and conduct nerve impulses from the CNS to muscles and glands.

The Peripheral Nervous System (PNS) may be subdivided further into a Somatic Nervous System (SNS) and an Autonomic Nervous System (ANS). The SNS consists of sensory neurons that convey information from cutaneous and special sense receptors primarily in the head, body wall, and limbs to the CNS and motor neurons from the CNS that conduct impulses to skeletal muscles only. Because these motor responses can be consciously controlled, this portion of the SNS is voluntary.

The ANS consists of sensory neurons that convey information from receptors primarily in the viscera to the CNS and motor neurons from the CNS that conduct impulses to smooth muscle, cardiac muscle, and glands. Since its motor responses are not normally under conscious control, the ANS is involuntary.

The motor portion of the ANS consists of two branches, the sympathetic division, and the parasympathetic division. With few exceptions, the viscera receive instructions from both. Usually, both the divisions have opposing actions. For example, sympathetic neurons speed the heartbeat while parasympathetic neurons slow it down. Processes promoted by sympathetic neurons often involve expenditure of energy while those promoted by parasympathetic neurons restore and conserve body energy.

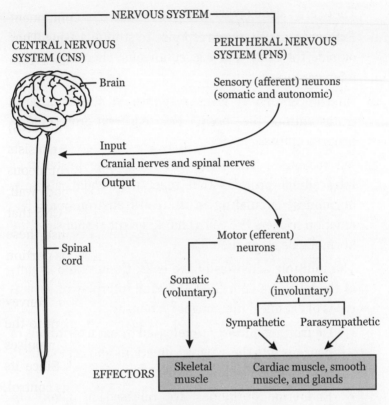

Fig. 15.1: Divisions of Nervous System

Receptors

The sensory, i.e. afferent nerve fibers terminate in the periphery as bare unmyelinated endings or in the form of specialized capsulated structures called receptors. The receptors give response to the stimuli. When the receptors are stimulated, a series of impulses are produced and transmitted through the afferent nerves. Thus, the receptors are biological transducers which convert various forms of energy, i.e. stimulus in the environment into action potentials in nerve fibers.

There are various types of receptors as:

1. Exteroceptors: It gives response to stimuli arising from outside the body. For e.g. cutaneous, chemoreceptors, telereceptors.

2. Interoreceptors: It gives response to stimuli arising from within the body. For e.g. visceroreceptors, proprioceptors.

3. Cell receptors: These are cell membrane proteins or intracellular proteins that react with chemicals (e.g. hormones) circulating in the cell's environment. The reaction triggers the cell's characteristic response to the hormone or other chemical.

The multiple activities of the cells, tissues, and organs of the body are coordinated by the interplay of several types of chemical messenger systems:

- Neurotransmitters are released by axon terminals of neurons into the synaptic junctions and act locally to control nerve cell functions.

- Endocrine hormones are released by glands or specialized cells into the circulating blood and influence the function of cells at another location in the body.

- Neuroendocrine hormones are secreted by neurons into the circulating blood and influence the function of cells at another location in the body.

- Paracrines are secreted by cells into the extracellular fluid and affect neighboring cells of a different type.

- Autocrines are secreted by cells into the extracellular fluid and affect the function of the same cells that produced them by binding to cell surface receptors.

- Cytokines are peptides secreted by cells into the extracellular fluid and can function as autocrines, paracrines, or endocrine hormones. Examples of cytokines include interleukins and other lymphokines that are secreted by helper cells and act on other cells of the immune system.

The endocrine hormones are carried by the circulatory system to cells throughout the body, including the nervous system in some cases, where they bind with receptors and initiate many reactions. Some endocrine hormones acts on entire body like the growth hormone and other at on specific target tissues, because only these tissues have receptors for the hormone. Example, Adrenocorticotropic hormone (ACTH) acts on adrenal cortex to secret adrenocortical hormones and the ovarian hormones have specific effects on the female sex organs as well as on the secondary sexual characteristics of the female body.

Integral membrane proteins can also serve as receptors for water soluble chemicals, such as peptide hormones, that do not easily penetrate the cell membrane. Interaction of cell membrane receptors with specific ligands that bind to the receptor causes conformational changes in the receptor protein. This in turn enzymatically activates the intracellular part of protein or induces interactions between the receptor and proteins in the cytoplasm that act as second messengers, there by relaying the signal from the extra cellular part of the receptor to the interior of the cell. Thus, integral proteins across the cell membrane provide a means of conveying information about the environment to the cell interior.

Thus, the receptors play an important role in multiple cellular functions like metabolism, hormonal activities and cell defense including cell death programming. Lack of oxygen in the intra cellular structure can only be noticed by these cell receptors.

The mechanism of action of the receptors with an example of thermoreceptors is explained in the following chart.

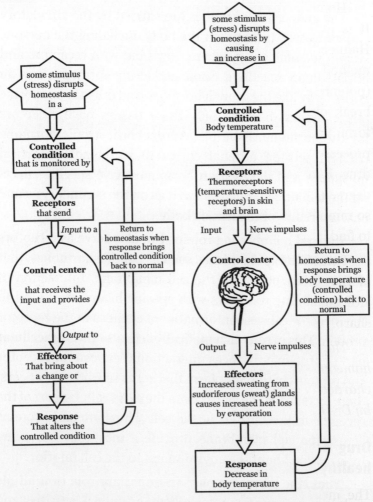

Fig. 15.2: Mechanism of transmission of impulse through receptors

Fig. 15.3: Thermoregulation of body through thermal receptors

Method of preparation of dynamic medicine

Today's scientific research and technology has nano-science as one of its main field. The development in this science facilitates the acceptance for molecular and micro-molecular sciences.

Homeopathic medicines are extremely minute molecules. It is impossible to count them even in nanometers. Dr Hahnemann has successfully put forth an outstanding method of preparation of Homeopathic medicines (potentization). The process of dilution and succession break down the medicinal particles to micro molecular form, which has a tremendous medicinal potential. These processes preserve the finest medicinal potential of the drug. Each and every finest micro-molecule carries highest degree of medicinal properties. The medicinal particles are so minute that even nano-science can't stretch out enough to find it.

Potentization in every step enhances the properties of the medicine. Once the medicine is prepared by the Homeopathic method, the molecule becomes strong and sharp.

The medicinal potential cannot be destroyed and hence homeopathic medicines have no expiry date. These special characters of medicine make it dynamic medicine as said by Dr Hahnemann.

Drug proving / Action of homeopathic medicine on healthy human being

The medicinal properties of homeopathic medicines are preserved in the alcohol. The alcohol or globules are the mediators to carry the potentized form of homeopathic medicines.

The action of the homeopathic medicine starts with the intake of micro-molecular dose. When the prover takes (by mouth) the first dose of the potentized medicine, the globules starts dissolving in saliva and initiates its action by stimulating the nerves of the mouth, tongue along with olfactory nerve, simultaneously through the receptors.

1. Corda tympanic fibers of facial nerve.

2. Glossopharyngeal nerve.

3. Vagal nerve.

4. Olfactory nerve.

In fraction of seconds the mouth receptors are stimulated with the micro-molecular substances of the homeopathic medicines.

Various receptors relay the information about micro medicinal molecule via, facial, vagus, glossopharyngeal and olfactory nerve to the cortex.

The cerebral cortex analyzes the received information. Analyzing occurs by different pathways in the CNS and both at conscious and subconscious level.

After knowing the properties and characters of the medicinal component, cerebral cortex and hypothalamus initiate their appropriate actions.

The cerebral cortex as a leader gives the information to the various parts of CNS and through them, the information pass to peripheral nervous system. Via the dendrites of peripheral nerves it reaches to the cell through the receptors. Then the respective changes take place in the cell.

Receptors carry on the action according to the character of the regarded medicinal molecule e.g. Increase or decrease in the secretion of concerned gland.

The received message makes changes in internal and external environment of the cells for a particular duration.

It creates dysfunction in cell organelles especially mitochondrial dysfunction for specific period of time (temporary). Once mitochondrial functions are disturbed symptoms start appearing in the prover.

Every medicinal substance has its own individual characteristic symptom group and preferred location i.e. sphere of action.

e.g. Chelidonium majus acts on liver.

Antimonium tartaricum acts on lungs.

The medicine shows a generalized action not only on the specific locations but also on receptors of cells of different organs.

Action of Homeopathic medicine on diseased person

Our human body is a systematic organization of cells, tissues, organs and systems made up with various minute constituents (cell organelles, proteins, fats, carbohydrates, vitamins, minute receptors, etc.).

Energy required for functioning of every single cell is obtained from metabolism in mitochondria and there are various minute receptors guiding this process. Slightest disturbance in any of the process in mitochondria will lead to cell damage.

The basic dysfunction being at such a micro level, cell requires a medicine which will carry out correction at same level. So the dynamic potential of Homeopathic medicine is only capable to reach such a minute level and bring out the repair and reconstruction.

In order to establish health and to get all organs to its optimum function, proper oxygen supply is a necessity. Homeopathic medicine works for the same purpose. Via receptors and CNS it shows its action on the cell organelles especially mitochondria. It stimulates the mitochondria to utilize more oxygen molecules and to reestablish the aerobic metabolism required for proper functioning and defense mechanism of the body. Thus, the abnormal function of cell can be brought back to normal with the properly selected Homeopathic medicine.

This is the dynamic action of the Homeopathic medicines. It is the most rapid and gentle way of healing.

The discovery of 'law of similar' is based on fundamental principles. Accordingly, the dynamic disease can be treated with medicinal substance having similar micro molecular properties. As per the nature's law two similar diseases can't stay together and the stronger one (potentized medicine) will remove the weaker (disease manifestations) and will reestablish health. Later on the potentized medicinal properties will gradually disappear by dynamic body reactions.

Importance of Vital Force (Oxygen)

Importance of Vital Force (Oxygen)

As we review the book, we realize that there are several misconceptions about Vital Force. Different names are put forth by the stalwarts and eminent homeopaths, like electro-dynamic force, simple substance, supernatural power, spiritual power etc. which do not give any comprehensible meaning. All these concepts create great confusion for homeopathic physicians especially the budding homeopaths. While explaining the homeopathic philosophy Dr Hahnemann mentioned that vital force plays a central role in health, disease, and cure and presented this idea very well. But due to lack of scientific explanation for the concept it resulted in varied definitions and theories of vital force and the misleading journey started from these different views.

The modern medical science will never accept any vague explanations about the concept of vital force because every science is based on scientific laws, principles, and proving.

The newly developing nano-technology and molecular science are accepting the existence of extremely minute substances. Still new things are being added in cellular and physiological functions. So, one can come to the conclusion that there are lots of things yet to be learnt.

So, this book is an attempt to explain the concept of vital force scientifically.

The Vital force is a solid foundation for explanation of Homeopathic philosophy.

One of the various misconceptions about vital force is to believe that it is soul and others believe that it is the mind which is the central force for curing the sick. They try to look at the sick person through the mental symptoms. The question then arises that, what is the importance of physical generals? How the physician is going to know about different kind of sensations, thermal conditions, the location, modalities, and directions of physical generals which are of prime importance for prescription. Is Dr Hahnemann's proving method faulty? Why did he include the physical generals, the peculiar and characteristic symptoms in his drug proving and materia medica? Why didn't he add only the mental symptoms which are the very easiest way to come to the conclusion of the sick person's mental state? What is the importance of totality?

So if physicians rely only on mental symptoms, it will be the one sided prescription. There will be no scientific justification for the given prescription and also there will be a big doubt regarding the process of cure.

Many physicians are thus going off track because of this baseless practice which is in vogue through books and seminars. This is very misguiding concept as to how the law of 'Similia-Similibus-Curentur' will be followed after giving importance only to the mind symptoms?

The answer to these questions is to follow only Hahnemann's concept about totality of symptoms which includes the characteristic symptoms, sensations, thermals, physical generals and the mentals.

After reading this book, one will come to the conclusion as to what is exactly curable in the sick, to remove the disturbance in the body at cellular level; we need to remove the central disturbance (i.e. oxygen) which is the only cause of the disease.

As mentioned earlier, every cell consists of the receptors which act as a well organized cellular maintenance system. They carry the various information to and from the CNS which helps to carry out the numerous functions of the body. The defensive action of receptors can also be noticed in the sensitivity to surrounding environment. The receptors are sensitive to the slightest stimuli which creates disturbances leading to cell injuries like ischaemia, infarct, necrosis, metabolic disturbances, and toxins which enter the human body including bacteria, viruses, and allergic substances.

Homeopathic medicine act on the cellular receptor system. Accordingly there are dynamic but temporary cellular oxygen energy disturbances created by artificial medicine which is responsible for manifestation of peculiar signs and symptoms of that particular medicine. The receptors identify the artificial disease producing power which is responsible for drug proving.

Oxygen plays a generalized role in every cellular function including the biological aerobic process. The lack of oxygen creates disease and abnormal sensations in the human body which are recognized by CNS through receptors. Therefore, healthy and harmonious state of body demands appropriate oxygen supply.

Thus, by summarizing this new scientific concept about vital force, I would like to conclude, making a firm statement that, *Yes! 'Vital force is nothing but oxygen energy'.*

I would like you to recall the 10th aphorism related to vital force as described by Dr Hahnemann, in the similar manner as I have mentioned i.e. the material organism, without the vital force (oxygen), is capable of no sensation, no function, no self preservation; it derives all sensation and performs all the functions of life solely by means of the immaterial being (the vital principle) which animates the material organism in health and in disease.

I owe my gratitude to Dr Hahnemann who liberated this science of homeopathic philosophy and removed the darkness of the medical world with the help of **'Similia Similibus Curentur'.**

Bibliography

1. Text Book of Medical Physiology 11th Edition – C.Guyton, & John E. Hall, [Published by: Elseveir, a division of Reed Elsevier India Pvt. Ltd., 17-A/1, Main Ring Road, Lajpat Nagar – IV, New Delhi – 110024, India.]

2. Human Physiology – Dr C.C.Chatterjee.(Part-I) [Published by: A.K. Chatterjee. For and on behalf of Medical Allied Agency, 13/1B Old Ballygunge 2nd Lane, Culcutta – 700019]

3. Essentials of Medical Physiology 2nd Edition – K. Sembulingam & Prema Sembulingam. [Published by: Jaypee Brothers, Medical Pulblishers (P) Ltd. B-3 EMCA House, 23/23B Ansari Road, Daryaganj, Post Box 7193, New Delhi 110002, India.]

4. Harsh Mohan's Text Book of Pathology, 4th edition. [Jaypee Brothers, Medical Pulblishers (P) Lts. B-3 EMCA House, 23/23B Ansari Road, Daryaganj, Post Box 7193, New Delhi 110002, India.]

5. Principles of Anatomy & Physiology - Tortora & Grabowski. 8th Edition. [Harper Collins College Publishers.]

6. Harrison's 15th Edition: Principles of Internal Medicine Volume 2 - Eugene Braunwald, Anthony S. Fauci, Dennis L. Kasper, Stephen L. Hauser, Dan L. Longo, J. Larry

Jameson. [McGraw-Hill, Medical Publishing Division., USA.]

7. Mosby's Paramedic Textbook, 3rd Edition – Mick J. Sanders. [Published by: Elseveir, a division of Reed Elsevier India Pvt. Ltd., 17-A/1, Main Ring Road, Lajpat Nagar – IV, New Delhi – 110024, India.]

8. Organon of Medicine, 6th edition – Samuel Hahnemann. [Published by: B. Jain Publishers Pvt. Ltd. New Delhi – 110055]

9. 'The Genius of Homeopathy – By Stuart Close [Published by: B. Jain Publishers Pvt. Ltd. New Delhi – 110055]

10. Kent's -Lectures on Homeopathic Philosophy – By Dr J.T.Kent [Published by: B. Jain Publishers Pvt. Ltd. New Delhi – 110055]

11. 'The Principles and Art of Cure by Homeopathy' - By Dr Herbert Roberts [Published by: B. Jain Publishers Pvt. Ltd. New Delhi – 110055]

12. The Science of Homeopathy - By George Vithoulkas

13. Text Book of Obstetrics – D.C. Dutta. [New Central Book Agency (P) Lts. 8/1 Chintamoni Das Lane, Calcutta 700009]

14. Website: www.encyclopedia.com